MOTHER NATURE'S BABY

*THE ESSENTIAL BABY GUIDE
OF NATURAL CURES
&
CHEMICAL FREE LIVING*

**BY
DIANE KIDMAN**

Mother Nature's Baby
by
Diane Kidman

Copyright © March 19, 2014 by Diane Kidman

All rights reserved. No part of this publication may be reproduced, stored in a retrieval system, or transmitted by any means – electronic, mechanical, photographic (photocopying), recording, or otherwise – without prior permission in writing from the author.

Printed in the United States of America

Cover Design by: Diane Kidman

Cover Photo by: Ann Troast Photography

Published by: carp(e) libris press, LLC

Visit the author website: http://www.DianeKidman.com

Table of Contents

Introduction 5

IMPORTANT: When to Seek Medical Help 10

An Antibiotic Alternative for Baby 13

Allergies & Asthma 17

Breastfeeding & Promoting Lactation 30

Cold & Flu 46

Colic 55

Constipation 63

Coughing 68

Cradle Cap 73

Diaper Rash 79

Diarrhea 91

Ear Infection 97

Eczema 104

Fevers 108

SIDS 113

Sleep Solutions 118

Teething 130

Why Organic? 138

The Question of Soy 140

Proper Baby Nutrition 146

Baby Food by Age 151

Homemade Baby Food Recipes 160

Baby Food Variety - Creating Your Own Combinations
.... 169

Finger Food Ideas 174

Freezing Baby Food 179

Cleaning With Baby in Mind 183

The Impossible Task of Clean: Organizational Tips .. 201

Natural Beauty for Mom 206

Natural Skin Care & DIY Health Products 208

A Final Word 217

Bibliography 219

About the Author 221

Introduction

The first time my baby caught a virus, I did what I do best: I panicked. It was obvious he was uncomfortable, which made me an even bigger mess. Crocodile tears rolled down his face, and this sweet baby who hardly ever raised a fuss had turned into a puddle of feverish sobs. I was new to the whole natural parenting thing; the whole parenting thing in general, actually. And so with the best of intentions, I drove to the pharmacy. Scanning the shelves, I was ill prepared for what I discovered. Every box and bottle I picked up instructed me not to give it to my son until he was at least two years old! But my baby was sick now.

Had he waited for his first illness until he was two, we'd have fared no better. Artificial colors and flavors, sweeteners, high fructose corn syrup, and preservatives peppered every ingredient list. And let's not even get started on the side effects, the sorts of things that cause teenagers to drink them for fun. It was disheartening, frustrating, and anger inducing. Not a single item was available that day for my six-month-old with a fever and a stuffy nose.

Chances are that if you're reading this, you're as frustrated as I once was. Congratulations on already searching out the answers to natural baby care! Perhaps you know a smattering of herbal medicine for yourself, or maybe you enjoy essential oils or organic produce. But transferring that sort of lifestyle onto a baby can feel rather intimidating, even dangerous.

That's where this book comes in. We'll be talking about remedies and homemade products you can make yourself with herbs, essential oils, and common items you already have in your kitchen. We'll also discuss everything from baby nutrition (including homemade organic baby food) to homemade housecleaning products and even a few beauty products for mom.

These pages will not only give you and

your growing family peace of mind, but it won't drain your wallet. Turns out many homemade products and natural remedies are big money savers. The house cleaning products alone will save you a bundle.

Why Alternative Medicine?

In early 2007, the Centers for Disease Control and Prevention revealed a study that showed in a two-year timespan, over 1,500 babies and toddlers were taken to emergency rooms due to bad reactions to OTC (over-the-counter) cough and cold medicines. Three babies died. As it turns out, many of these emergency room visits occurred because worried parents broke down and gave their little ones medications not intended for babies under the age of two years.

It may sound a little scary giving an infant or young child herbs or natural remedies. But if you're careful and gather a little knowledge, you'll soon find there are remedies that are safe and gentle enough for our tiniest of family members. You'll be able to relieve their symptoms with minimal to no side effects, and you'll feel great about doing it naturally. Herbs are often cost effective, too. A bag of bulk chamomile, for instance, can be very inexpensive and last a long time with proper storage; and there are so many ailments that can be treated with just that one herb, as you'll soon find out.

In fact, since there are so few OTC medications available to babies and young children, I think you'll be surprised to find that, with just a few herbs kept at the house, you can alleviate problems that can't be handled with a trip to the pharmacy. You'll feel more in control over your baby's health, and all it takes is a bit of knowledge under your belt.

Here We Go!

Alright, now that you're all geared up for learning about cures, remedies, and natural baby and child care, let's get started. Remember, this is just the tip of the iceberg.

There are centuries of remedies out there to discover. As your little one grows, you can grow your own knowledge and continue to heal your child as naturally as possible.

IMPORTANT: When to Seek Medical Help

You're about to embark on learning natural remedies for your baby, and while that is a wonderful and rewarding experience, it cannot ever be the only thing you rely on for baby's health. If you ever feel that parental itch that tells you something just isn't right, DO NOT HESITATE to go to a trusted doctor, ever. Always check with your doctor first before administering any medications, natural or otherwise. If you have the least misgiving about an herbal or natural remedy, ask! Always ask. Learning natural remedies is one of the best things you can do for you and your family, but there is no substitution for the input of a trusted physician when it's warranted.

While I am trained in herbalism, I am not a doctor. My remedies are suggestions and are not meant to replace medical treatment in cases of serious illness. If treating your baby as naturally as possible is important to you (and I hope it is), make sure your pediatrician is on board with your views and has some knowledge of alternative medicine and proper nutrition. It's alright to interview a doctor first, to ask around for recommendations from friends, to change doctors when you feel you're not seeing eye to eye. But always make sure you have a trusted doctor you can go to.

If your baby doesn't respond to home treatment; if he's three to six months of age and showing signs of serious illness with a high fever of 101°F or higher, six months or older with a fever of 103°F or higher; or if your baby is under three months and has any fever at all; or if he's lethargic, weak, unresponsive, or difficult to wake, get medical treatment immediately. If there are recurrent ear infections, or if there are any visible red streaks on the skin from any point of infection, if bug bites or bee stings seem to be giving an allergic reaction such as excessive swelling, difficulty breathing, or unresponsiveness, seek medical attention immediately.

If your baby has dry lips and the inside of the mouth is dry, or if there has been a drop in the usual number of wet diapers, this is a sign of possible dehydration. Seek medical attention.

In newborns, if the fontanel (also known as the "soft spot" on the baby's head) is swollen, go to a doctor immediately. This is a possible sign of meningitis.

An Antibiotic Alternative for Baby

Many of the issues we'll be discussing in this section of the book could lead to an antibiotic prescription from the doctor, so let's start out with learning an alternative. It's one I've been using since my own childhood, and so it was a no brainer for me when I had a child. Shortly after my baby's umbilical cord stump fell off, I noticed it looked a bit red and irritated. So I did what any first-time mom would do: I called the pediatrician convinced my child was in peril of having a misshapen bellybutton for the rest of his life. The doctor asked me to bring him in so she could take a look. She told me it was just fine, and that the slight redness was nothing to be worried about, so long as I cleaned it regularly and kept an eye on things. But just to be safe? She wrote me a prescription for an antibiotic.

I never had that prescription filled.

Antibiotics Aren't Always the Answer

Every day, parents take their children to the doctor's office hoping to leave with a prescription for an antibiotic. But the U.S. Centers for Disease Control and Prevention have been urging doctors for several years now to lessen the frequency of antibiotic prescriptions. With so much use, more and more antibiotic-resistant bacteria are coming onto the scene. And also with so much use, we ourselves are becoming resistant to antibiotics. So what's an alternative we can use with our babies when the need to fight infection arises?

Acidophilus

Nature has provided us with something: probiotics, the exact opposite of antibiotics. Probiotics increase the number of beneficial bacteria in the body, whereas antibiotics kill off all bacteria, both good and bad. The probiotic we're discussing here is called lactobacillus acidophilus. Acidophilus is the good bacteria that makes yogurt, well, yogurt. When taken, it multiplies in your digestive tract and replaces our own bacterial flora. With enough of these guys around, things like sinus infections, yeast diaper rashes, and thrush have no choice but to disappear. They are also capable of reducing inflammation and improving immune function. Antibiotics, on the other hand, kill not only the bad bacteria but the good bacteria that naturally occurs and should remain in our bodies.

What's It Good For?

Babies can benefit from acidophilus in a myriad of ways. Any infections such as ear, lung, skin, yeast (including diaper rashes and thrush, a mouth infection some babies get); intestinal issues like constipation and diarrhea; and digestive issues such as gas, indigestion, and even colic. Acidophilus is the powdered form of the good flora that are in our guts and intestinal tracts naturally. But sometimes we don't have enough of these, so offering the acidophilus is an excellent way to boost the good bacteria we need for a healthy system.

Administering Acidophilus to Your Infant

To give acidophilus to an infant, Dr. William Sears recommends making a paste of the powder form of acidophilus with water or breast milk and rubbing it on the infant's gums once a day, or putting a teaspoon of the powder in a bottle once a day if you bottle feed. You can also take it yourself if you're breastfeeding, thus passing on the probiotic to baby.

There's no question antibiotics are sometimes very necessary and even life saving, but lactobacillus acidophilus is an alternative that is safe and effective; your baby won't build up a tolerance, and there are no nasty side effects. A health decision you can definitely feel good about!

Allergies & Asthma

The Centers for Disease Control and Prevention released a study in 2013 that states food allergies have increased by 50% in children from 1997 to 2011! That's a whopping spike in a short period of time, and there are no clear-cut answers as to why this is happening in developed countries around the world. There is much speculation, and I tend to side with those who put some blame on what we're eating and how it's grown. While we will talk about the importance of eating clean, healthy food in more detail later, let's cover a few things on allergies, both from food and from the environment, and what can be done to reduce allergic reactions.

Allergies are symptoms of an oversensitive immune system, and researchers are unsure as to why one person has allergies and another does not. So while I can't tell you how to cure your baby of all allergic reactions, I can give you some hints on how to alleviate the symptoms when they appear.

Pets

Pets are a common cause of allergies, so we'll start there. I'm allergic to cats myself. I have no pet cats these days because it's just too much sneezing and eye rubbing for my taste, but I grew up with cats. They took up residence in our home before anyone realized I was allergic, so when I started sneezing and wheezing from allergies and asthma, my parents took me to the doctor. Our family doctor wasn't one to mince words. He said, "Get rid of the carpet. Get rid of the drapes, the bedding, the stuffed animals, the cats." In other words, get rid of every homey comfort and creature and toy I loved. My parents weren't about to give away my beloved cats or toss my stuffed animals out. But they did tell me I could no longer sleep with the cat in my bed. In fact, the cats could no longer set so much as a paw in my room. No longer could I rub my face in their bellies, and if I played with them, I was to wash well afterward. No rolling in cat hair, no letting my favorite stuffed bear ride any kitty backs.

Granted, if allergies or asthma are very severe, you'll have to make some tough decisions. But even with several small changes, you can take a new look at the way many things are done in your house. If you know allergies and asthma tend to show up in your family tree, you can give babies a boost toward health right from the beginning.

Breastfeeding, Formula, and Solid Foods

According to the Generation R Study done by the Erasmus Medical Center in The Netherlands in 2011, feeding your baby only breast milk for the first six months can reduce their risk of developing asthma in early childhood. Breast feeding is great for babies whose families are prone to not just asthma, but allergies and eczema as well.

If you do choose to nurse, be mindful of what you eat and drink. The properties of your diet are often concentrated within the breast milk and passed to the baby. For instance, if you tend to drink a lot of cow's milk, your baby will receive the proteins within that milk which are difficult for him to digest. Peanuts contain another tough protein for babies to tolerate. If you suspect your baby is having allergic reactions such as rashes, eczema, or a stuffy nose, it is well worth it to catalog what foods you're eating. A diary of daily foods can help you figure out when baby has outbreaks and when she doesn't.

If formula is your only option, choose a hypoallergenic one, preferably one that's labeled as extensively hydrolyzed, as opposed to partially hydrolyzed, which isn't technically hypoallergenic. Research shows partially hydrolyzed formula makes little to no difference for babies with food allergies.

Watching the diet is important for babies experimenting with solids, too. Hives, congestion, eczema, and other such allergic reactions could be coming from food. Keep a daily diary of foods your baby eats and try eliminating anything you think might be a culprit, at least for a week or two. If things clear up, you can reintroduce the foods, one at a time, and carefully monitor your baby's reactions.

Smoking

While we've all heard it a million times, it must be said again and again: Never smoke around babies or children. Studies have repeatedly shown that when your child gets older, he'll get sick more often if he's been around secondhand smoke. His lungs won't grow as much as other children's, and bronchitis and pneumonia will be more common. Wheezing, coughing, and asthma attacks are more common for children who've been subjected to secondhand smoke, too. They get more ear infections, have more fluid in their ears, and are more likely to end up with tubes in their ears. If you have friends or relatives who smoke, ask them to smoke outdoors and not in your home or in your car or anywhere near your baby. Just opening a window and blowing the smoke through the screen isn't good enough. Ask smokers to wait awhile after they've smoked or to change clothing before holding your baby. Remember, your child's health is infinitely more important that the feelings of friends and family.

Indoor Allergens & Triggers

There are many possible allergens within the home, and eliminating them or controlling them can go a long way to staving off allergy and asthma attacks. Reduce your home's allergens by vacuuming at least once a week. When you vacuum, make sure babies and children are not in the room. Cover all bedding and crack open doors or windows to help ventilate the area, and don't allow any babies or children into the room until at least an hour after vacuuming. This allows the dust a chance to settle; because no matter how powerful the vacuum cleaner, no matter how great the filtration system, at least some dust will become airborne while you clean. Dust afterward by using a damp cloth and never use spray cleaners for the removal of dust. (You can check the Cleaning With Baby In Mind section of this book for natural DIY furniture polishes.)

Make a good assessment of what's in your child's room. Remove whatever dust catching items you can, or keep them impeccably dust free if you can't remove them; carpets, ruffled bedding, and curtains all hang onto dust like magnets. Stuffed animals do too, and you can vacuum them off with the hose and an attachment to remove as much dust as possible. Avoid using wool blankets or synthetic pillows, and purchase allergy-free bedding. Wash bedding weekly in hot water (130° Fahrenheit) and don't air the bedding outdoors if your child has allergies to pollens. You can also use allergy proof nylon or plastic coverings on mattresses and pillows to avoid dust mites; those little guys can cause all kinds of sneezing and wheezing.

Keep doors and windows closed between 5 and 10 a.m. if pollens are an issue, too. That's the time when pollens are heaviest and settling.

New carpets and furniture are usually prone to heavy outgassing. While there are some hard-to-find manufacturers that make formaldehyde free products, the average dresser, for instance, could outgas for several years after manufacture. And carpet can be pretty heavy on the VOCs. These chemicals are linked to numerous acute health conditions like asthma, nausea, even cancer and respiratory disease. This can make creating a baby's room tricky and redecorating the house an asthma reducing nightmare. I've gone through it myself, both in creating a chemical free baby room and in eliminating asthma and allergy triggers for the sake of my own health. If my family does purchase new furniture, we try not to get anything with particleboard since the glue that bonds it together is where most of the formaldehyde is. Solid wood is always best when possible, and if you can finish it yourself with a non-VOC varnish or sealant like paint, all the better. Another great option is gently used furniture. Of course, be extra careful with cribs and make sure they're sturdy, not more than a few years old, and within regulation. But buying used means it's already outgassed, and as is my experience, you'll often end up with a much higher quality for a fraction of the price of new. Spending time on a website like Craigslist is enough to turn one away from ever buying new again!

  Not everyone can afford a solid wood crib made by the Amish and finished with beeswax. So if you're completely stuck with a new piece of furniture containing particleboard, you can try using a product such as Safecoat Safe Seal, which is a synthetic product made to block formaldehyde emissions from particleboard. Zinsser Bull's Eye Shellac is another alternative. It's from a natural source (the lac bug's secretions after eating a certain tree sap), and while there are alcohols added into the shellac, those will outgas rather quickly. Just make sure that if you use it, you apply it in a well-ventilated area and wait at least 10 days before bringing the furniture into the house.

If you're in love with carpet, finding some that's VOC free can be about as easy as teaching your baby to play Bach for the upcoming church concert. While the CRI (Carpet and Rug Institute) claims that carpet actually traps allergens and is therefore healthier for you than hardwood, I'd rather not have any allergens trapped on the floor at all. Call me fussy, but I've lived with new carpet, old carpet, and hardwood floor and tile. Hands down the easiest floors to keep clean and allergy free have been the hardwood and tile. We installed prefinished hardwood so we didn't have to have varnish fumes indoors, and we asked the installer to nail it together so no glue was used. (That's where a lot of the stink comes from with new carpet and hardwoods.) I vacuum the hardwood floors which does a great job of trapping dust and debris; much more thorough than just sweeping, and it's faster, too.

Clean that Air

Now that all the perpetrators have been removed, you'll want to add a few things to improve air quality. We've all heard houseplants are a great way to scrub the air, and while I've seen a myriad of lists suggesting one type of plant over the other (Wikipedia has an interesting and extensive list), the bottom line is that all plants clean the air to some degree.

The leaves of your average houseplant absorb the chemicals in the air (they all have their specialties) and take them into the tissues and down to the root system. The chemicals are then turned into plant food. Another way plants transform toxic chemicals is by pulling air down around the root system while moisture is released from the leaves in a process called transpiration. It's one of the reasons why we live so harmoniously with plants, and why we can't do without them.

It is recommended that you place one houseplant per 100 square feet of living space.

When choosing plants for a child's room, it's especially important to make sure the plants are safe and not poisonous. A few good air cleaners on the "safe" list would be: spider plant, ficus, golden pothos, gerbera daisy, Chinese evergreen, and Mauna Loa. I like hanging baskets that can be kept well out of reach, regardless of a plant's safety. Because toddlers like digging in dirt. A lot.

If you're considering an air purifier, use one with a HEPA filter. HEPA stands for "high-efficiency particulate air." What that means for you is that tiny particles such as pollen, dust mites, pet dander, and tobacco smoke are trapped within the filter as air passes through it. My all-time favorite air purifying system would be anything from IQAir. Yes, they're pricey. But if you can afford it, nothing beats the quality. If you get a portable unit, be sure to keep it in the room where you spend the most time. If baby has allergies, then the baby's room is probably where you'll want it to be. Keep up on changing any filters when needed.

Creating a healthier environment for children who suffer from asthma and allergies does take some work and commitment, but in the long run, it makes a big difference. It's important not to feel overwhelmed with the task, and don't get down on yourself if you discover you've been doing something wrong all along. The best thing to do is to make the changes one at a time and move on. Remember, moving toward a chemical free lifestyle is a journey — not an instantaneous hop.

Breastfeeding & Promoting Lactation

What are the Benefits of Breastfeeding?

Glad you asked. Whether you're expecting a baby or you're already nursing a little one, it's good to know the benefits of breastfeeding. Some of us are still making the decision, some of us need encouragement to keep on going, and still others of us just like to be reminded from time to time how breastfeeding is nature's way of helping baby develop strong health. Here are a few facts on breastfeeding from La Leche League.

- Breastfeeding only (without additional formula) for the first six months of life lowers the risk of obesity.

- It lowers the risk of ear infections, viruses, diarrhea, chest infections, asthma, and other illnesses, even after weaning.

- There are long-term cognitive benefits. Breastfeeding for eight months or more results in higher verbal and performance IQ scores in seven- and eight-year-old children.

- It decreases the risk of childhood diabetes.

- It makes baby's potty more regular (and less stinky, I might add), and it puts off that first virus longer. When the first virus does occur, it's shorter.

Don't forget the benefits to mom, either! For the nursing mother, hormones are released that calm her. What a great help in the beginning stages of motherhood! The food is free, compared to the high cost of formula. It's already heated, it's totally portable, and there are no late-night trips to the convenience store because – oops! – there's no more formula in the house and baby's hungry NOW.

Let's not forget to mention the faster weight loss for mom. Breastfeeding burns at least an extra 500 calories a day. That means for the duration you choose to breastfeed your baby, whenever you take seconds at the dinner table, you're allowed to say, "What? I'm breastfeeding."

Getting Started

If you're about to be a first-time mom, breastfeeding can seem a bit scary, and that's okay. You're not alone. Our generation didn't grow up seeing breastfeeding very often, and for many of us, the first time we see it up close will be the first time we feed our newborn babies. That was my case. I was in the hospital surrounded with nurses who didn't know anything about breastfeeding. I certainly didn't. And the lactation specialist wasn't due to visit me until the next day. So I tried and tried on my own to get my baby to latch on, but he wasn't getting it and neither was I. The nurse I had in the first hours after my delivery was frustrated, both with me for wanting to breastfeed, and with my baby for not being a good "first-timer." I'll never forget her solution to introducing him to the breast: shove his head at it. Oddly, this did not work. She left my room more anxious than ever, and I heard her plain as day outside my open door talking to another nurse. She said, "Do you know how to breastfeed? I got a mother in there who insists on doing it, and I don't know anything about it." I wasn't sure what she was doing in a maternity ward, and I would have assumed she was filling in from another department, but the nurse she asked didn't have anything to offer, either. So I was left to tough it out alone.

The next day the lactation consultant came while I had visitors in my room, a lovely couple who drove a long distance to see me and my new baby. When the specialist asked to see how it was going, I glossed over it and said it was fine. I was embarrassed to talk about it in front of my visitors, even more embarrassed to ask them to leave. Had I known they were perfectly comfortable with the situation and had watched all their grandchildren breastfeed, I wouldn't have cared. But I was new to things and nervous.

When my baby still refused to eat much, the nurses came in with a bottle of sugar water. I cringed, but they made me scared that he wasn't gaining weight, so I relented. Fortunately, a doctor came to check up on me and said not to worry. He told me the very best thing for me and my baby was to go home, get comfortable, and spend alone time just being together. "No pressure," he said. "You'll be surprised what getting out of this hospital and into your own home will do for the both of you."

He was right. It took just a few hours of being home and in the nursery before we got the hang of things. And instead of losing weight, my son grew by leaps and bounds.

I said all of that to say this: If you've decided to breastfeed and it seems alien to you or uncomfortable, or if you're afraid you'll fail, don't sweat it. Find a good lactation consultant. Talk to friends who have done it. Get on some online forums and some websites like La Leche League's excellent forum. And keep a hotline number handy, such as 1-877-4-LALECHE. It's important to realize that breastfeeding happens "naturally" for very few of us in the beginning. But once you figure it out, nothing seems more natural. Nothing on earth.

Traditional Chinese Medicine for Lactation

I enjoy studying Traditional Chinese Medicine (TCM). My husband sometimes comes home to things like black fungus soup and sesame tea, and even stranger things have shown up in his stir fry, all so I can see what it does to us when we eat it. A major part of Chinese medicine is food that cures and heals. When you're nursing or pregnant, you have to watch those medications. But if it's healthy food used to heal you, those concerns will lessen.

If your problem is lactation, TCM has that one covered, and I'm speaking from personal experience. My experiences in breastfeeding were pretty normal, I think. It took us some time to figure it out in the beginning like with most new moms, but we did it. After several months of established routine, I had one day when I seemed a little more — er — productive. My eight-month-old, eating his usual large amounts, wasn't able to keep up with my output. If you've ever breastfed, you know that's an odd turn of events. Knowing that foods can affect lactation, I wondered what I'd eaten.

This was right after we'd started eating some different things due to a new TCM manual I was reading. So naturally, I knew in my case, it had to be a dietary change I had made within the last 24 hours. I looked up the foods in my book, Chinese Natural Cures by Henry C. Lu, PhD and narrowed it down. For me, it had been the tofu. But I learned a lot more about foods for lactation in the process.

Normally, a woman's lactation will be up and running three or four days after she gives birth. But if it isn't, Dr. Lu suggests in his book, Traditional Chinese Medicine, several foods that can help. He explains that there are two different types of lactation problems. In the first case, a woman may experience little or no milk secretion or clear, diluted milk. This woman would have no swelling or pain in the breasts, pale complexion, poor appetite, and fatigue. For her, some foods recommended would be beef, chicken, lettuce, peanuts, red date, and tofu.

If a woman is experiencing a total absence of milk or only a little bit, swelling and painful breasts or hardness, and if she has concentrated and sticky milk, Dr. Lu suggests different foods, including: beef, button mushrooms, sweet potatoes, and sweet rice.

Of course, you don't have to have those issues to reap the benefits of these milk producing foods. As I stated earlier, tofu did it for me. I had it in stir fry and some soup. (If you're not into tofu, try scrambling some eggs and adding tofu cubes at the end, cooking until the tofu is heated through. You'll hardly notice it's in there. Sprinkle some shredded cheese on it for a high protein breakfast.) If one of the items doesn't seem to work for you, try another one, or combine them. Imagine a beef stir fry with green onions and tofu. That would have to be good! Be creative with your combinations. Have fun with it. Let's face it: Eating is a lot more fun than using a breast pump to stimulate lactation.

Herbal Teas

Since the beginning of herbalism, women have been turning to tea for a help in boosting lactation. There are several to choose from, so you can pick your flavor. And if one doesn't do it for you, go ahead and try another. Always purchase the freshest tea you can find. If you go to a health food store and find a dusty box of lactation tea on the back of the shelf, it might be too old and not work for you. I like bulk herbs because they're cheaper and it's easier for me to see and smell the herb before I buy it so I know I'm not getting a bag of ancient sawdust. As long as it's been stored out of direct sunlight, is in a sealed container, and the clerk doesn't use her hands to fill your bag, you've got a good chance of getting effective herbs. If you're buying from a store and not online, smell it and make sure it's fragrant. Even if you're not sure what the herb is supposed to smell like, it should smell like something more than weak hay. If you purchase from an online retailer, make sure they're reputable. I like Frontier Co-op, Mountain Rose Herbs, and Starwest Botanicals.

Fennel is a popular lactation tea and is particularly good for women having lactation issues due to stress. Not only is it effective for both milk production and colic relief, it has a pleasant licorice flavor. What you'll usually find for fennel teas will be the seeds, but leaves and flowers work too. Steep a teaspoon of seeds in nearly boiling water for 10 to 15 minutes. Drink two to four cups a day. If you're pregnant, check with your doctor before using it.

Fenugreek tea is another good choice. Prepare the tea by steeping a teaspoon of the seeds in nearly boiling water for 10 or 15 minutes. (But if you're pregnant, fenugreek should be avoided.) One cup of tea taken two to three times a day usually increases milk flow noticeably within 24 to 72 hours.

Alfalfa tea is helpful for more than just increasing lactation. For moms who went through a rough labor or had a Caesarian section, it's good for convalescing, as it helps you recover. It's highly nutritious and loaded with minerals, and it boosts your calcium absorption, so it adds health benefits to the milk. Prepare a standard infusion by steeping a teaspoon of the flowering herb in a cup of nearly boiling water for 10 or 15 minutes. Two or three cups of tea a day should be sufficient. If you're pregnant or if you're prone to lupus, don't take alfalfa tea.

Dill is another herb that has multiple benefits for a nursing mom and her baby. It not only stimulates lactation, it's good for tummy upset and colicky babies as well. So when you drink it, your baby can get relief from colic through your supercharged milk. Make a standard infusion of the dill seeds by steeping a teaspoon in nearly boiling water for 10 to 15 minutes and drink it two to four times a day.

Breastfeeding While Sick

Being sick is bad enough, but when you have little ones relying on you, you need to get healthy quick! If you're pregnant or nursing, you're unable to take most over-the-counter medications as it is. And if you're like me, you'd normally rather not deal with those over-the-counter side effects either. I got a crash course in treating illness the natural way through a nasty bout with the flu when my son was about six months old. In an attempt to get better as quickly as possible, I put many of my old tricks into practice and learned some new ones, as well.

First things first: If you feel the slightest onset of a cold or flu, kick start your health. Lemons are a great source of vitamin C, and when your body is fighting off illness, vitamin C is used up more quickly. Try half a lemon in a full 16-ounce glass of water about four times a day. (You should be drinking lots of water anyway.) If taken at the very beginning of a cold, or even if you think you've just been exposed, you can often nip that virus in the bud before it even gets a chance to set in.

If you can't knock a fever, try this little trick: Garlic. Garlic is often referred to as Russian penicillin. Raw is always best, and I know you can get it in tablets, but garlic in its whole form is always the most loaded with the healing properties you need. If you can get a hold of organic garlic, all the better. I know, I know. It's stinky stuff. But you're sick and probably won't be going anywhere, anyway. You can nibble one clove alongside you dinner. If you don't want to offend your family, have them eat a little too. Not only will they no longer be offended by your smell, they'll be building up their own immunities as well, and they'll have a better shot at not catching your virus. I've heard some concerns about the flavor of the garlic getting into breast milk, but I've also heard some babies really like it. It certainly can't harm your baby, or there'd be a lot of unhappy

Italian bambinos out there.

Got a sore throat? The lemon and the garlic will help, but if you still need more of a kick, don't forget the old-time remedy of chamomile tea with honey. (Or just a teaspoon of honey can soothe the throat and a cough, too.) If you have green tea around, try that. It's loaded with so many health benefits they're too many to number here.

If you're feeling stuffy, take a good snort of salt water. Some sea salt mixed with purified water, as strong as you can handle, will help clear out the sinuses. If you're prone to sinus infections, this can aid in keeping a cold from turning into an infection later. You can use a neti pot (follow the instructions in the box) or sniff some water from an eyedropper. Gargling warm saltwater is also a great way to help a sore throat and kill infection.

Don't forget to eat the hot stuff! (Check with your doctor on this one if you're nursing or pregnant — not everyone agrees with spicy food during this time.) It may initially make your nose run even more, but nothing can clear the sinuses like some jalapenos or hot mustard. Capsaicin, the stuff that makes hot peppers hot, also has the power to release endorphins, something we could all use more of when we're under the weather.

For sinus infections, turn towards yogurt. The live cultures in yogurt are a natural antibiotic and will fight off that nasty infection. For a tasty way to take it, mix a cup of the yogurt with a cup of blueberries and ½ cup water or cow's milk. Run it through the blender for a healthy smoothie. (The blueberries are loaded with countless beneficial properties as well. They're great for diarrhea, constipation, and urinary tract infections, not to mention the power to sharpen your thinking and memory.)

If you're pregnant, nursing, or just plain unable to keep up with kids while doped up on cold capsules, try these natural remedies for what ails you. You'll be pleasantly relieved.

Aid for Dry, Cracked Skin

Many nursing mothers experience dry, cracked skin, even bleeding, at the nipples. This can make breastfeeding feel a bit like medieval torture instead of a blessed bond. If this is your problem, you can try soothing the dry skin with coconut oil or olive oil. Massage onto skin between feedings, before bed, and whenever you can. Both oils are incredibly healing and safe for you and your baby. Be sure to keep your skin clean, but without using soaps or lotions, especially scented ones. Believe it or not, your breast milk has antibacterial properties, so applying a bit to the cracked area can help, especially if baby has thrush, which is a yeast infection that sometimes occurs in the mouth. This infection can be passed on to you, so keeping clean and using fresh breast milk on the area can reverse any infection you might have picked up.

Cold & Flu

A baby's firsts are joyous occasions when everyone makes goofy faces and claps and fusses as if baby has discovered nuclear fission. But a first cold doesn't get such a warm reception. The morning my son woke up with his premiere case of the sniffles and a hefty cough, I was thankful that he was able to hold out until almost six months of age; but somewhere deep inside, I was hoping he'd just never get a cold.

Incidentally, most children get between six and ten colds a year. For those in daycare or school, they can get as many as 12 per year! That's an awful lot of tissues and tea. It's good to get a handle on natural remedies now because there will be more in the future; the following remedies are good to use not only in baby's first year, but for years to come.

Is it a Virus?

If your baby has a cold, he'll probably have a runny nose with clear mucus in the beginning. (The mucus will most likely thicken and turn yellow, green, or gray as the cold progresses.) A cough might be present, as well as a low-grade fever, but the fever will generally show up sometime after congestion sets in. The flu is something that usually hits hard and fast, and includes a fever, diarrhea, and/or vomiting. Allergies, on the other hand, present with watery, itchy eyes and a runny nose with clear mucus that doesn't change color. Sneezing fits and hives or itchy skin that last weeks or months at a time are another sign it's allergies and not a cold. Also, allergies don't produce a fever.

Go Homeopathic

As I mentioned in the beginning, I was more than disenchanted with the great void of cold and flu medications for babies. So when I finally came to the realization I had to stick with the natural way of doing things, I decided I'd better pack us up and take a trip to my local health food store. Due to a great experience with homeopathic teething tablets (lo and behold, they worked; read up on that in the Teething chapter), I just had to go see what they had for colds.

I found a whole line of homeopathic tablets, and I was happy to see they had many choices for colds and flu. The bottle I found only gave instructions for age one year old and up, but the health store consultant reassured me that homeopathic tablets are safe for all ages.

Another bit of advice I was given is in regards to nursing mothers: If your nursing baby has a cold, remember to eat the healthy foods you'd eat if you were the one with the cold. Try the remedies from the Breastfeeding and Lactation section, including lemon water and fresh garlic.

I always kept a humidifier with a little reservoir for inhalants in the baby's room. I still do this, no matter who's sick in the household.

Putting a few drops of eucalyptus in the reservoir, I'd let the baby play in the room or take his nap. It's surprising how fast this can work with little ones. I do advise not leaving a baby in an enclosed room with the eucalyptus oil, however. It can sometimes be too potent if you're not careful. Keep the door cracked open and stay with the baby to monitor the strength. Remember, they're more sensitive to smells than we are. And always keep essential oils out of their reach.

Lemony Stuffy Nose Relief

Boil four cups of water with ¼ cup dried lemon thyme, remove it from the stove, and help baby inhale the steam. For little ones, use very close supervision and inhale with them. Then you'll be certain the steam isn't too hot or too powerful. Or try ½ cup apple cider vinegar and ½ cup water. Boil and inhale the steam, same as with the lemon thyme concoction.

The Salt Water Cure

One of the most helpful remedies for the stuffy nose is salt water. This can be used for any age, and it doesn't have to be uncomfortable. For infants and toddlers, you can try a product called Baby Simply Saline. As the name implies, it is simply water and salt in a container that makes it easy to spray into baby's nostrils. It's a gentle mist, so it's not uncomfortable; and since there's nothing but water and salt in it, you can use it as needed. No preservatives, no stinging. Try using this a good 15 minutes before feeding your baby to help ease the stuffiness and make eating easier.

The Breast Milk Cure

If you're nursing a newborn, an unusual but effective technique is to put a few drops of breast milk into each nostril with an eyedropper. Sounds weird? Well, since the breast milk has bacteria fighting properties, it's actually a great natural choice. And it's free!

That's Horseradish

When an infant's nose is severely stuffed, it makes eating difficult if not impossible. Herbalist Ed Smith told me about this horseradish trick that will clear a newborn's nose when nothing else seems to work. To do this, you'll need some freshly ground horseradish. You can find a horseradish root in the produce section of most grocery stores. Ground horseradish in a jar will probably be less potent, but if that's all you can get, it's worth trying. Just make sure it's pure horseradish and doesn't contain other ingredients. Place a spoonful of the ground horseradish in the palm of your hand and gently cup your hand over your baby's mouth and nose, being careful not to completely block airflow. Allow your baby to get a few inhalations of the fumes, then take your hand back. You can repeat this until baby sneezes, which is likely to produce a large mess, so be prepared for it!

Herbal Tea

If your baby is older than six months of age, you can prepare a weak cup of chamomile tea. It will relax her, help her sleep, and ease some of those cold and flu symptoms. Steep ½ a teaspoon of chamomile in a cup of nearly boiling water for about five minutes, then strain. You can put half the tea in a bottle and serve it when it's cool enough to drink. Save the other half for later. Remember, don't sweeten the tea with honey until baby is at least one year old. You can also use the colic seed tea recipe from the Colic chapter, if there are any stomach issues present with the virus. The herbs in that combination are quite beneficial for several cold and flu symptoms.

Soothing a Dry, Irritated Nose

If baby's nose gets dry, crusty, or irritated due to all the sneezing and wiping, you can apply some of the homemade diaper ointment I'll show you how to make in the Diaper Rash chapter. Just make sure that you've never "double dipped" in the container during diaper changes, or use a separate container of the ointment set aside for this purpose.

Sleep Positions

While it may be tempting, it's never a good idea to prop your baby up for sleep to allow for better breathing. Adding pillows or cushions to the crib to help baby sit up can cause suffocation hazards. And while some recommend putting baby to sleep in a car seat, the seats aren't approved for such use. It might be okay for nap time if you're around to monitor your baby, but avoid using that as a nighttime solution.

When to See a Doctor

Babies who have a high fever should see the doctor. Call your pediatrician's office to see what his recommendation is, and what he considers to be a high fever, since different doctors go by different guidelines. In general, if your baby is under three months and has a fever of any sort, you should call the doctor. Babies three to six months of age should see a doctor if the fever is 101°F or higher. Babies six months and older should go when the fever hits 103°F. If a fever lasts more than two days, no matter how old your baby is, call the doctor. Babies with excessive coughing or wheezing should also see the doctor, as should babies who pull at their ears, especially while eating, or who cry when put to bed (if that's not their normal bedtime style). Keep a close watch on your baby for anything unusual or out of the ordinary. I know that's tough — babies seem to change every day as it is, but if you feel red flags being raised in your parental radar, it's better to be safe than sorry.

Colic

Nothing can try the patience of a new mom and dad than a baby with colic. You dream of quiet evenings rocking a peaceful baby to sleep, and instead you have a squirming, screaming newborn who just can't get calm and comfortable. Thankfully, there are ways to help colicky babies find some peace, giving mom and dad a chance to enjoy their little bundle.

Colic is characterized by lots of crying, what seems to be abdominal pain, and irritability. This usually starts around one month of age and continues through about four to six months. Colicky babies tend to cry from one to four hours at a shot, have high-pitched, loud, continuous cries, and often pull their legs toward their stomachs or push the legs straight out. They clench their fists, they grimace, and they even hold their breath. Sometimes they have flushed faces and cold feet. If your baby typically cries for three hours or more, three times a week for three consecutive weeks, that's a good indication it's colic. Be sure to talk to your pediatrician about it so you're sure it's colic and not something else, like an ear or bladder infection, two other things that can cause a lot of crying.

There's good news and bad news about colic. The good news is, it usually goes away when the baby is six months old. The bad news is, it usually goes away when the baby is six months old. That's an eternity for an exhausted family. At least there's a long list of natural things you can try to alleviate the pain everyone's feeling about now.

Herbal Teas

Steep one teaspoon chamomile (dried) and one teaspoon fennel seed in one cup of boiling water for 15 minutes, covered. Add about ½ tablespoon of the well-strained tea to your baby's formula or some pumped breast milk. You can use this up to three times a day if needed.

If you want to get a little more complex about your remedies, try this colic seed tea: Mix together two tablespoons each of dill seeds, fennel seeds, and anise seeds. To that mixture, add two tablespoons catnip and two tablespoons chamomile which helps to relax the baby. Add teaspoon of your herb mixture to a cup of boiling water and cover it to steep for about 15 minutes. Strain out the herb very well and mix some with an equal amount of water. Give the baby some of this diluted tea from a bottle between feedings. (Just a few swallows, though. It shouldn't replace a regular meal.) Nursing moms can take the tea themselves and pass it to baby that way; but don't take the tea if you're currently pregnant.

Herbal Baths

Adding calming herbs such as lavender flowers, hops, lemon balm, or linden flowers can reduce spasms and quiet your baby. Make an infusion of herbs by preparing a cup of tea. You can add the tea directly to the bath. About a teaspoon of herbs steeped in a cup of nearly boiling water for 15 to 20 minutes should do the trick.

Mom's Diet

No, I'm not going to give weight loss advice here. But if you're nursing, the cause for the colic could be on your dinner plate. It's possible that avoiding foods such as dairy, caffeine, spicy foods, garlic, or the gassy vegetables of the cabbage family might help baby's digestion. Rule them out one at a time. You can also try adding a good acidophilus supplement to your diet. Acidophilus helps aid in digestion and if it's in you, it'll be in your baby. Ultimate Flora by New Life is an excellent brand, as is Garden of Life's Primal Defense.

Homeopathic

Homeopathic tablets are very safe, and many parents find them quite effective. While you should be able to find a good selection in your health food store or online, homeopathic remedies are showing up in standard pharmacies and grocery stores more often all the time. Just be sure to follow the product's directions closely, even though homeopathic remedies are generally safe.

Chiropractics

My cousin's second baby had a horrible case of colic. After trial, error, and many sleepless nights, they decided to try taking her to a licensed chiropractor experienced in dealing with babies and colic. The chiropractor was able to massage the baby's abdomen and make some gentle adjustments. The transformation was so impressive the father eventually changed career paths. He's now a chiropractor!

Music Therapy

Sometimes the sounds of relaxing music can help baby through the tough days and nights of colic. Try lullabies, classical music selections for babies, and CDs with heartbeats and womb sounds. Another favorite would be ocean sounds since the crashing waves are similar to what baby heard in the womb. (My son's favorite was a Sting CD called Songs from the Labyrinth. It involves lots of beautiful, calming music and Sting reading quietly from the letters of John Dorland.) If you're away from your music selection, try singing or making a gentle "Shhhh" sound in baby's ear.

Motion

An old popular way to soothe baby is motion. Car rides, stroller rides, and rocking are all tried and true for many a crying infant. If the weather is pleasant, go outside and get some fresh air while holding your baby. Keeping your baby in your arms can be stress relieving and comforting for him. If you need your arms free, invest in a good baby sling or carrier. And don't forget to let someone else have a try at holding the baby. Remember, you're going to need frequent breaks in a quiet corner if you're going to have the patience and the will power to get through colic.

Heads Up

If you're breastfeeding your baby, try having her sit up a bit more when eating. Also, make sure there's a good latch with no loud sucking sounds. For bottle feeders, make sure the nipple is set in the bottle correctly and that your baby isn't sucking air with the milk or formula. If you are using formula, make sure it doesn't include any cow's milk, as this can cause upset. Burping your baby is especially important for the colic prone.

Read Up

One good bit of advice is to pick up The Happiest Baby on the Block, a book by Dr. Harvey Karp. If you can't fathom reading through a book right now (and who would blame you?) there is a DVD as well. Dr. Karp helps parents learn how to swaddle their babies and comfort them, giving them the sense that they're still in the womb, a place he says newborns miss. My son didn't have colic, but we did swaddle him and use Dr. Karp's techniques after a kind doctor in the hospital where I delivered highly recommended the book.

Don't Give Up

Colic is indeed a frustrating challenge. But the good news is, it doesn't last forever. In the meantime, try these helpful remedies, and don't forget to treat yourself with some relaxing teas and time out for both mom and dad. Letting baby spend time with grandma for an afternoon doesn't make you a bad parent; just a relaxed one.

Constipation

It's difficult not to become obsessed with what's in our baby's diapers. Let's face it, their systems are different than ours, they go potty in a myriad of colors, and sometimes a baby can go a week without a bowel movement and be just fine! While most breastfed babies have a movement at least once a day and formula fed babies go once a day (sometimes more), there's a huge variation here. Some babies go several times a day like clockwork, then stop. Others, you're just happy to see something in the diaper once or twice a week. So how do you know whether or not your baby is constipated?

What Should It Look Like?

A baby's poop comes in a virtual rainbow. But for the most part, breastfed babies make a mustard poop: yellow with specks. Formula fed babies tend toward tan, yellow, and green poops.

But if your baby varies from this spectrum, don't be alarmed.

When Is It Not Okay?

If there's mucus, blood, or water present in the poop, take your baby to see his doctor. This could be a sign of an allergy or an infection. If it appears hard and solid, it could be a sign of constipation. A constipated baby will also often have a hard, distended stomach. It's also possible for a constipated baby to pass what looks like diarrhea in the diaper; but this could just be some liquid getting around a blockage in the intestines. So if his output looks less than usual, despite what appears to be diarrhea, it could still be constipation. One key to deciphering whether or not it is constipation is whether or not your baby is going less that his usual amount, no matter what that usually is. Also check to see if any stool that is being passed is hard or seems painful for baby to eliminate.

What Goes In...

While babies who are exclusively breastfed are rarely constipated, it does happen. If you breastfeed, watch what you're eating. It could be causing constipation or diarrhea in your baby. If constipation is the problem, try avoiding dairy cheese, wheat, eggs, and refined or processed foods for a while. (If you're breastfeeding, avoiding the refined and processed foods are a good idea in general.) Be sure to take in plenty of fresh fruits and vegetables, and always drink plenty of water. This will help regulate baby, whether the issue is constipation or diarrhea.

If your baby is on formula and has a problem with constipation, it could be due to an iron fortified formula. Talk with your pediatrician about switching formulas.

If your baby is on solid foods, then be sure to add plenty of age-appropriate fresh fruits and vegetables to her plate. Drinking enough water is also important. A few foods that constipate are: rice (including rice cereal), bread, applesauce (due to the pectin), and bananas. Foods that relieve constipation include: plums, peaches, apricots, whole grains, peas, pears, spinach, and prune juice. Incidentally, switching your baby over to solid foods is often a cause for a bit of constipation, especially if baby was breastfed first. Breast milk is so easily digestible that sometimes the introduction of solids is a bit of a shock to the system.

Prunes Aren't Just for Grandma

For infants, constipation can often be cleared up by adding just a teaspoon of prune juice to a bottle of formula or breast milk. Be patient for it to work and don't give any more than one teaspoon in a day to avoid turning constipation into diarrhea. It's always good to check with your pediatrician before trying to correct constipation on your own; remember, a baby's schedule isn't the same as yours.

Movement to Create a Movement

And speaking of movement, to get the system going again, try laying baby on her back and gently moving her legs as if she's on a bicycle. Alternatively, you can rub her tummy clockwise around (but not on) the bellybutton. Oftentimes, these motions will encourage peristalsis, which is the wavelike movements the intestines make. Older babies can be encouraged to crawl a few laps around the living room.

When to Call the Doctor

If the belly is hard and distended, if there is vomiting with the constipation, and if there is frequent and/or painful urination, call your pediatrician right away.

Coughing

It's 2:00 a.m. Do you know where your baby is? Yes, you do. Because there's a wee little cough coming from her crib, and you've been sitting in her room wondering how on earth you can stop it. If over-the-counter medications make you queasy (and they should), there are several natural things you can try to quiet your baby and help her, and you, get a much-needed night of rest.

Humidifiers

Every baby's room should have a good humidifier. There are some great ones on the market at a variety of price ranges; make sure yours is one you can easily take apart and clean yourself. Also, make sure it doesn't require any fancy-shmancy chemicals in the humidifier water. It's a little counterproductive to set up a humidifier to help the air quality and have it misting out chemicals meant to defeat buildup in the filtration system. Try to find a humidifier with a special removable reservoir for drops. Steer clear of any store-bought concoctions; for we will make inhalants ourselves!

Pure, high-quality essential oils can be purchased at varying prices, but whether they're expensive or not, one thing is for certain: One tiny bottle can last you a good long time. Only two to three drops are needed in the reservoir. (Don't mix the drops directly into the water tank.) There are several oils you can try. Eucalyptus, thyme, sage, peppermint, and rosemary are my favorites. Once you have the humidifier up and running, keep the bedroom door propped open and check in on baby periodically. The air should never be heavy with the smell of the oil. You yourself might find more relief from a stronger aroma, but for a baby's sensitive nose, it can be overwhelming.

Steam Baths

Steam can be used to loosen a tight

cough. Take your baby into the bathroom with you and close the door. Run a hot shower and sit in the bathroom for 10 or 15 minutes, allowing him to breathe the steam. Or fix baby a warm bath and let him splash around a little. For a more calming effect, you can try mixing a cup of chamomile tea into the bathwater.

Herbal Tea

And speaking of herbal tea, babies over six months of age might try a mild mixture of sage and thyme tea. Steep one teaspoon of a blend of the two herbs in a cup of nearly boiling water for about 10 minutes. Make sure the tea isn't too strong; give it a taste test yourself first. As long as the tea doesn't replace an all-important breast milk or formula feeding, it can be a very helpful remedy.

Simple Massage Oils

Vapor rubs like Vicks is too harsh for your baby. It is also a petroleum based product, and any product containing petroleum is never a good idea for any age. Instead, try mixing this ointment: ½ teaspoon dried ginger, 1 teaspoon olive or sweet almond oil. Rub it on baby's chest, either night or day. Another option is to massage coconut oil onto your baby's chest. It's soothing, gentle, and feels good when the lungs are aching from all that coughing activity. The third option, garlic oil, doesn't go on the chest; it goes on the feet! An old remedy that does work, you can prepare your own garlic oil by chopping four cloves of garlic and putting them in a glass jar with ¼ cup of olive oil. Stir it, then put the jar in a pan with some water, then allow it to simmer on very low heat for about 20 to 30 minutes. Let the oil cool, then strain out the garlic. Take a small amount of oil, perhaps ¼ teaspoonful, and massage it into the bottoms of your baby's feet. Cover with socks that you don't like, because they'll never be the same again.

When to See the Doctor

If your baby is three months old or younger, you should always see the doctor when coughing occurs. For severe cough or infection, consult your doctor. For babies three to six months old with a fever of 101°F or higher; or babies six months and older with a fever of 103°F and up, see a doctor. Wheezing, difficulty breathing, and the appearance of any blood in coughed up mucous are also reasons to set up an appointment right away.

Cradle Cap

Around my house, we always referred to this scaly condition as "cradle crap." Those flaky little crusty pieces of skin clinging to your baby's otherwise perfect head and/or eyebrows can be annoying. It usually shows up by three months of age and can occasionally last into the toddler years. What is that stuff, anyway?

No one seems to agree on what causes it: hormones from mommy, reactions to an immature digestive system, the list goes on. One thing experts do agree on is it's not due to bad hygiene. At my son's three-month appointment, my pediatrician assured me it wasn't dangerous. It rarely gets to be an extreme case, and most babies aren't bothered by it at all. Mostly it's just an annoyance to parents who are constantly flicking little flakes out of baby hair. (Never peel them off, by the way. That can cause infection.)

Olive Oil

There are some natural and safe ways to deal with cradle cap if you are tired of waiting it out. One way is to rub a little olive or vegetable oil onto your baby's scalp and put a hat on him. Wait a few hours or overnight, then take an infant's hairbrush or a soft toothbrush and gently brush the scalp. I tried olive oil on my son and it did help. But washing it out was a real bear. If you attempt this, use a very small amount. I wouldn't recommend treating the cradle cap with added essential oils, however. Babies can be too sensitive to the smells and properties, even developing lifelong allergies to those particular herbs if they're overused.

Aloe Vera

Aloe vera gel is another solution. That, too, can be rubbed into the scalp and left on, same as the oil. It washes out cleaner. Just be sure it's out of the way of baby's reach so she doesn't eat it. The juice of the aloe plant contains latex, which can cause irritation of the intestines resulting in diarrhea. If your baby is allergic to latex, she'll probably be allergic to aloe vera too.

Chamomile Tea

A good strong cup of chamomile tea can be of help, as well. Prepare a strong cup by steeping one heaping teaspoon of flowers in a nearly boiling cup of water for 20 to 30 minutes; strain, cool, and apply with a cotton ball. A word of caution: While it's not common, some people are allergic to chamomile, usually the same people who are allergic to ragweed. Testing a bit of tea on the inside of your baby's arm is advisable before applying it to the scalp. If no reaction shows after several hours, you should be okay. If your baby's cradle cap seems to be bothersome or itchy, the chamomile can bring relief. Alternatively, comfrey root tea can be used as a rinse after regular shampooing. Prepare the tea ahead of time, just as you would the chamomile. As a final rinse, pour the comfortably lukewarm tea over the scalp and gently massage in. Don't rinse it out; just towel dry and air dry the rest of the way.

Glycerin Soap

When I first started using glycerin soap, I started seeing improvement on the cradle cap almost immediately; I was noticing no new buildup on my son's scalp, but the old buildup was still there. Afraid to scrape at it because it might hurt or cause infection, I was sort of hoping it would start coming out on its own during washings and combings. That didn't happen — until I found a finer baby comb. (Note: I didn't try to remove what was still attached to his scalp; only what was caught at the base of his hairs. Remember, picking it off isn't advised.)

The comb I began using had small closely-spaced teeth that, when I combed his hair, simply lifted off the old cradle cap buildup. I couldn't believe how much came up from his scalp from one combing. I washed his hair first to soften the scalp, towel dried until his hair stuck up like a baby orangutan, then gently combed his hair. I repeated that the next day, and to my surprise, his scalp was beautifully clean with nary a scalp crud to be found.

On the "don't" side of things, make sure you don't use dandruff shampoo or adult shampoo on your baby, and avoid irritating or strong soaps. Those are too harsh and can bother the scalp rather than soothe it. Most of all, don't fret. It is a condition that usually clears up with time; most babies outgrow it by their first birthday.

However, if you notice any puss or crusting, or if it looks tender and irritated, check with your pediatrician. It can occasionally develop into an infection, or it may be an indication of something more serious.

A Final Note: I am sorry to say liquid glycerin doesn't always work so well on adult hair. Imagining my own locks to resemble my son's gleaming tresses, I dumped some on my head and scrubbed away. When my husband returned from work, he took one look at my new do and asked, "What happened to you? You look like a shrub."

Diaper Rash

Every baby experiences it: a red, irritated bottom caused by doing what babies do in their diapers. It can be anywhere from mildly uncomfortable to tear-inducing burning whenever baby urinates or makes — well, the other stuff. The market is loaded with all sorts of lotions and creams to take the sting out and clear up skin, but if you're going the natural route, these options probably don't rise to your standards. That's okay. You can fix the problem yourself!

First of all, you must know that there are two main types of diaper rash. We have the run-of-the-mill red bum, sometimes with little bumps and even some bleeding if it's worse. Then we have the yeast rash. This one is recognized by its raised red marks, usually more concentrated in the area of the genitalia and going back towards the bottom. The more common of the two is the first one.

There are many things you can do to clear up the average diaper rash. Several of the following remedies are also great forms of prevention. It may take a little experimentation to figure out which of these works best for your baby.

Change Diapers Often

Rashes are commonly caused by what your baby put in his diaper to begin with, so clean, fresh diapers are a good way to reduce the risks. Change a newborn's diapers at least once every two hours; as urination frequency lessens as your child grows, you can change diapers less often. If baby already has the rash, urine or bowel movements can burn. After cleaning his bottom well, give him a moment to air dry. I used to put a diaper on my son without fastening it shut. Then I'd just talk to him or fix his socks until he had a minute to dry. Some parents swear by a hair dryer on a low setting, just to totally dry the bottom. They claim this trick alone can eliminate future rashes, as well. You can also leave the diaper off and lay your baby on his tummy for a few minutes while he dries off. A nice waterproof play covering on the floor would be a fun place for baby and parent to play while they await a fresh, dry behind.

Oatmeal Bath

One remedy I have used frequently is an oatmeal bath. I just used a little oat flour (you can buy it or run uncooked organic slow cook oats through a high powered blender until it's the right consistency) and sprinkled it in the bath water. Just a couple of tablespoons swirled in a warm bath eases the redness and calms irritated skin. This is also a great way to soothe other skin irritations or dryness.

Baking Soda and Water

Mix a small amount of baking soda into a cup of water, and wipe baby's bottom with the solution before putting on a clean diaper. Again, this is one where you'd want to make sure the bottom is nice and dry before diapering.

Aloe Vera Gel

I've noticed that a lot of aloe gels you buy at the store have all sorts of things in them with a smidgen of aloe to keep the plant's name on the bottle. Others have preservatives, which is understandable — it is, after all, the juice of a succulent plant. But what if you simply bought an aloe plant? These are so much cheaper than the gels. The gels with just a few ingredients are quite pricey, but an actual aloe plant is very inexpensive, it's a nice decoration for the kitchen (I use mine for all the times I burn myself cooking), and it provides fresh aloe vera gel whenever you need it. To use the plant, snap off the tip of a leaf (about an inch or so) and squeeze the jelly-like substance out on your finger. If there seems to be a lot of leaf left, you can save it in the refrigerator. Aloe can also be used on burns, cuts, bug bites, and sunburn. Just keep it out of reach of babies and young children, though. It can cause diarrhea. And don't use it if baby has a latex allergy.

Try Homemade Wipes

There are some good all-natural baby wipes out there that are made without alcohols, parabens, and other things many of us try to avoid, but nonetheless, the cost of wipes add up. If you're looking to do things on your own and save some money as well, consider making your own baby wipes. You can still enjoy the convenience of a disposable wipe if that is important to you, or you can make reusable wipes and save a bundle while you save the environment.

For either type of wipe, the cleanser formula I always used was the same. Just use one cup of distilled or purified water, about one tablespoon of liquid glycerin soap, and about one tablespoon of natural baby oil or olive oil. Shake these ingredients together in a jar or bottle with a lid. If you're going to be out for the day and don't want to lug dirty washcloths back home, you can cut a roll of bleach-free absorbent paper towel in half with an old bread knife. (Seventh Generation makes a nice unbleached paper towel.) Pull the cardboard rolls out of the middle and put the paper towel into a container with a lid. Pour the cleanser evenly over the paper towel. For reusable wipes, fold cotton baby washcloths into a stack (enough for one day at a time or they could mildew), and put them in a container with a lid. Pour over enough of the cleanser just to make sure they're all damp but not dripping. I used these two ideas throughout my son's entire diaperhood, and I never once missed store bought wipes.

Go With Cloth

There are a myriad of cloth diapers available these days, and in a wide range of prices and styles. While the initial cost to get started might seem steep, the difference between purchasing cloth diapers every once in a while to disposables every week or two is astronomical! If you're in the least bit of doubt, compare the cost of how many disposables you go through in a week (the average use is 2,300 diapers in the first year!) compared to a stack of cloth diapers. The numbers won't lie. And neither will that healthy baby tushie.

Vinegar Rinse

If you are going the way of the cloth diaper, you may want to alter the detergent you're using to wash the diapers. Or you can add some vinegar to the rinse cycle to alter the alkalinity in the wash, which helps a lot of babies get past the rash. About a half a cup of vinegar per load would be sufficient. (Incidentally, vinegar is also a nice fabric softener replacement. Check out the household cleaning section for more on natural laundry.)

Yeast Rash

If you think your baby has a yeast rash, there are a couple of things you can try. One of the best things for yeast is acidophilus. This is a good bacteria that is found in yogurt. You can buy probiotic diaper ointment or just get the capsules in the health food store (usually in the refrigerated section). Taking the capsules yourself if you breastfeed is a wonderful way to pass on the benefits to baby. You'll also reap the benefits yourself, as acidophilus is great for the digestive tract and acts as a natural antibiotic without killing the good bacteria we need. (If you want to give the acidophilus directly to your baby, you can find those instructions in the Acidophilus section of this book.) If your baby is eating solids and is at least eight months of age, a nice organic plain yogurt is a good way to get that healthy bacteria in your baby's system.

Cleansing baby's bottom with a calendula tea can also rid the skin of a yeast infection. Prepare the tea by steeping a teaspoon of the dried flowers in a cup of almost boiling water. Steep covered for 15 to 20 minutes, then strain out the herb. When the tea has cooled, you can apply it with a cotton ball. If you don't double dip, you can continue to use the tea throughout the entire day. Make a fresh batch every day until it's no longer needed.

One thing to remember: Yeast feeds off sugar. If you've ever made bread or baked with yeast, you know that often one adds some sugar and warm water to the yeast to activate it. The yeast in the body feeds on sugar, as well. So make sure baby isn't getting any sugar in her diet, and if you're breastfeeding, you may want to back off the sugary stuff awhile.

Diaper Ointment Recipe

While this recipe takes a bit of effort, it's well worth it. I swore by this recipe when my son was a baby because it worked wonders for reversing diaper rash. Combine ½ ounce of each: comfrey leaf, comfrey root powder, St. John's wort flowers, and calendula flowers. In a double boiler, combine one pint of olive oil with the herbs and steep on very low heat for two hours. Strain out the herbs and return the infused oil to the double boiler. Add ½ cup grated beeswax and stir to melt. (I like using a wooden chopstick.) If the oil has become too cool for the wax to melt, turn on a low heat once again.

Test the salve by placing a small spoon of warm mixture onto a plate. Allow it to cool (I put it in the freezer for about 30 seconds to a minute) and test the consistency. It should be thickened but easy to smear. If it's too runny, you can add more beeswax and test again. If it's too thick, try adding a touch of olive oil to the mix and test again.

Pour into a clean glass container with a large mouth and a tight lid. If you have dark glass, all the better. Either way, store it in a cool dark place. While the shelf life is different depending upon the climate in which you live and the freshness of the oil when you started, it should be good for several months to a year or more if stored properly. When the salve begins to smell like rancid oil, it's time to dispose of it and make a fresh batch. Do a nose test frequently. Hint: It's always a good idea to keep a couple of separate, smaller containers of the ointment, too. Set aside one for travel and one for other uses, such as an irritated nose during cold season.

What Not to Use

While the old standbys are often mineral oil or petroleum jelly, these two items are not only petroleum based and therefore unhealthy, they block the skin's ability to release toxins. And while they seem thick and moisturizing, the opposite can be true; either one can cause acne and dry skin. Also steer clear of talcum powder. The inhalation is harmful and can cause coughing, vomiting, even pneumonia. Instead, as long as you're certain the diaper rash isn't from yeast, you can use pure organic cornstarch or arrowroot powder. If you choose to go with cornstarch or arrowroot powder, keep it out of baby's reach, no matter how safe it feels. Babies like to play with containers and siblings like to imitate mommy and daddy, sprinkling powder on the baby. Any fine powder can be an irritant to the lungs, especially small baby ones.

Homemade Baby Powder

To make your own talc free baby powder, combine two parts white clay (Kaolin clay) with two parts arrowroot, ¼ parts slippery elm, and ¼ parts comfrey root powder. Mix it together and put it in a shaker bottle (like the salt and pepper shakers you have in your kitchen cupboards that you never use because the holes are too big and dump on everyone's food like a typhoon of black and white). Cover the top and shake well to combine ingredients. If you can find them, try adding ⅛ parts ground myrrh, ⅛ part powdered goldenseal, and ⅛ parts powdered echinacea for an extra boost. Cover and shake again until combined.

Diarrhea

Being obsessed with your baby's diaper output is a normal part of parenting. When things change from the usual, it can sound our parental alarm bells. For the most part, babies have ever-changing bowel movements. From how often they go (several times a day to only once a week) to how it looks (tan, yellow, green, and just about anything in between), it all becomes top priority discussion between moms and dads. I remember many a serious talk among groups of moms at play dates and get-togethers. I never thought I'd be one of "those" moms, but we all do it at some point. Here are a few tips that will not only relieve baby of his messy situation, it'll make you the star of the next baby storytime group when you pass on your newfound knowledge.

When Is It Diarrhea?

If your baby has watery bowel movements, goes much more frequently than usual, or goes more profusely than usual, it could be diarrhea. The most common cause of acute diarrhea is rotavirus, which usually resolves itself around three to ten days. Other common causes are: food sensitivity, viruses, bacteria, parasites, medication, or functional bowel disorders. While diarrhea is rarely great cause for alarm as long as baby is continuing to gain weight and eat normally, always consult your doctor when diarrhea is present, especially for infants and newborns. It takes only a day or two for diarrhea to dehydrate a young baby. Your pediatrician will be able to assess diet and environment, and will be able to make sure baby isn't becoming dehydrated.

Water

No matter the age of your baby, if you suspect diarrhea, make sure she's getting enough fluids. That means breast milk or formula. Most experts agree babies don't need supplemental water until six months of age. If there's diarrhea present, don't try to rehydrate baby with juice, especially apple, pear, or prune. If your baby is old enough to have juice, discontinue it until the stool has returned to normal. No colas, soft drinks, or bottled fruit "beverages" which typically contain no juice, just a cocktail of "natural" and artificial flavors, should ever be given to babies or toddlers.

Herbal Teas

If you are breastfeeding, you can drink some herbal tea yourself, thus passing on the medicinal qualities. Teas that are especially helpful in cases of diarrhea would be: meadowsweet, rosemary, or red raspberry leaf. For acute diarrhea, you can administer rosemary tea directly to baby until you can see a doctor. Gently simmer one teaspoon of rosemary in a cup of water for 15 minutes. Give baby a dropperful of the cooled tea every 15 minutes for an hour, then a dropperful ever one to two hours until the diarrhea is relieved. Rosemary works as an antispasmodic and an astringent; hence it's perfect for diarrhea.

What to Eat

Don't force the solid foods if your baby doesn't feel up to it. In fact, small meals are better during bouts of diarrhea. For babies old enough, the best foods at this time are those included in the BRAT diet: bananas, rice, applesauce, and toast. Babies on solid foods can benefit from these diarrhea-stopping foods. A mashed ripe banana, for instance, will help control diarrhea while replacing much needed potassium. Creamed brown rice blended with a bit of plain organic yogurt is another alternative. And remember, while applesauce can stop diarrhea, apple juice does just the reverse. So steer clear of apple juice for now.

Signs of Dehydration

Since dehydration can set in quickly

when diarrhea is present, you should know the signs. If your baby seems listless, irritable, and thirsty, has a decrease in the number of wet diapers (six wet diapers a day is normal for a baby), produces fewer tears when crying, has a dry mouth and his skin seems dry and less elastic, your baby could be dehydrated. At this point, doctors often recommend a rehydration drink. While things like Gatorade and Pedialyte are helpful, they also contain preservatives and artificial flavors and colors. It's quick and easy to make your own.

Homemade Rehydration Drink

For babies of any age, you can prepare your own rehydration drink instead of purchasing the brands at the store. Nursing babies should continue to nurse as usual; the drink can be given after usual feedings as a supplement. Combine 4 cups water with ½ tsp. salt (or ¼ tsp. salt, ¼ tsp. baking soda), and 1 to 1 ½ cups rice cereal for babies. Offer one tablespoon to one ounce of the mixture every 15 to 30 minutes; increase as tolerated. Alternatively, you can try this recipe from The Rehydration Project of the Centre for International Child Health Institute: Combine 1 liter purified water with 8 teaspoons sugar (molasses or raw sugar contain more potassium and may be better alternatives), and 1 tsp. salt. Dissolve the sugar and salt in the water, then add ½ cup orange juice and one mashed banana.

Ear Infection

One of the most common reasons for a trip to the pediatrician is ear pain. It occurs most frequently in children up to the age of eight years, and for many children, the problems start in that first year of life. Since a baby's head is not yet fully developed, it can cause bad drainage, thus an ear infection. Of course, you can't ask your baby if her ears hurt, but you can look for the telltale signals of ear pulling and crying, a fever that goes up at night and comes back down during the day, pus drainage, or a bloody discharge, and swollen tonsils or glands.

A middle ear infection is caused from the buildup of fluids when there's not enough drainage. With an increase of pressure, bacteria starts to grow; and if left to its own devices, it could result in a ruptured eardrum and permanent hearing loss. Such an infection is often brought on by colds, sinusitis, and an upper respiratory or throat infection. But it could just as likely come about from allowing your baby to fall asleep with a bottle, when the milk has the opportunity to pool up and drain into the ear.

Take Your Positions

Since the pain is usually greater while laying down, your baby might wake up crying. You can't prop her up on a stack of pillows at night, but you can put her in her car seat during nap time. Just be sure to supervise carefully, as car seats are not designed for indoor use or a crib substitute.

Garlic Oil

To make your own garlic oil, take about 4 cloves of garlic and chop them finely or run them through a food processor. I like to give them a few good whacks with the side of my cooking knife to release the oils. Make sure to use fresh garlic and not the pre-chopped kind in a jar from the grocer's, which may contain preservatives and additives. Place the garlic in a clean, dry glass jar and cover with about ¼ cup of fresh olive oil. Place the jar in a pan filled with water and heat it on very low heat in a double boiler for 20 to 30 minutes. (I fill a saucepan with water and set the jar in the middle.)

Once your oil has cooled, strain it thoroughly. You may now use a dropper to place a few drops of the oil into the ear. Hold it in place with a bit of cotton. It stays in better if one lays on one's side for a while. To remove the oil, tip the head gently to the side, catching the oil with an old clean towel. Wipe the surrounding area of the ear, but don't try to flush it out. Repeat as needed.

St. John's Wort Oil

As someone with sensitive ears myself, I understand the unbearable pain of an ear infection. While the garlic oil can reverse infection, nothing has ever attacked the pain for me like St. John's wort oil. I prefer to make it myself, but that requires gathering the bright yellow flowers of the plant in the wild during the last weeks of June through the beginning of July, then soaking them in a jar of olive oil for two weeks before straining the oil. You can certainly do that if you're confident you can properly identify the plant, and I recommend you give it a shot if it's at all possible because the oil is magnificent. But for most busy people with a baby (especially a baby with an ear infection), it's more practical to just buy some. Make sure the oil is pure, not expired, and has an orange-red to ruby red color. It should smell sort of lemony, not rancid. St. John's wort won't reverse an infection, but it knocks the pain out faster than you can say, "Why's my baby crying?" After warming the drops to body temperature by holding the bottle in your hand, apply just a drop or two into the ear canal, wait a minute, and then drain it back out by tipping the ear over a towel. I've used this on severe ear pain, and I feel instant, within-seconds pain relief. It's truly amazing stuff, and it's worth its weight in gold while you wait for the infection to clear. Note: Never use drops in the ear if the eardrum is ruptured or if fluid is present.

Acidophilus

While I recommend you get your baby to a doctor right away if you even suspect an ear infection, you can try acidophilus as an antibiotic alternative. See the section entitled An Antibiotic Alternative for Baby for detailed instructions.

You Are What You Eat

Make sure that if you've been giving your baby any cow dairy products like milk or cheese, you stop. The casein protein which is present in cow's milk is oftentimes associated with recurring ear infections. (Breast, rice, and nut milks are not, as these do not contain casein.)

A Little Ear Wiggling

You can sometimes pop your baby's

Eustachian tubes open with the following trick, which will allow for the drainage of fluid: Gently pinch baby's earlobe between your thumb and forefinger, then wiggle it. Carefully pull out and down a few times. This action can produce the same "pop" that happens when you yawn or swallow.

Clear Out the Nose

Using a light saline spray made for babies that contains only salt and purified water (such as Simply Saline Baby Nasal Relief), spray each of baby's nostrils and then gently suction the nostrils out using a baby nasal aspirator. Sometimes this will stimulate the fluids within the nose, thus clearing the Eustachian tubes.

Find the Root Cause

If an infection is recurring, it's important to track down what's causing it. Is it diet? Is it sleeping with a bottle? Sinus issues or allergies? A nutritional deficiency, such as not enough zinc or omega 3s? Talk this over with your pediatrician and try to get to the bottom of things before resorting to something like having tubes put in (called a tympanostomy), which is standard practice for recurring ear infections. If tubes are brought up by your doctor, do your research well. Recent studies show the risks outweigh any benefit that may be had.

Eczema

What on this earth is sweeter than your baby's face? You could stare at your son or daughter all day. And although all babies are perfect in the eyes of their parents, there are issues that sometimes need a little healing, such as dry skin and eczema. Newborns are especially prone to dry patches of skin on the cheeks, and even on the scalp, arms, and legs. Fortunately, most babies outgrow eczema. But what do you do in the meantime?

What Is Eczema?

First, it's important to understand what eczema is. It's a skin condition that, in babies, most often shows up as dry, patchy, flaky skin that can be red and irritated. It most often will show up on baby's cheeks or on the arm and leg joints. When babies get eczema, it's frequently because of a lack of ceramides, which are the fatty cells that protect the skin, so when baby doesn't have enough, the skin gets dry. It can be hereditary, and while most babies will outgrow it, a few will not. In general, it's not caused by allergies; but certain things can trigger it or cause it to grow worse, such as soaps, perfumes, fabrics (especially wools and man-made fabrics), dust, and a lack of humidity. Stress, heat, and sweat can also cause eczema to grow worse. And while experts still haven't agreed on whether or not food has any part in it, some believe things such as dairy, peanuts, and eggs should be avoided.

Vitamin E

My son battled with small patches of dry skin on his chubby cheeks for the first two or three years of his life. I tried every natural solution I could come up with, but I was surprised to discover this most simple of solutions: vitamin E.

You know those cute little amber vitamin E capsules? They can be cut open and squeezed, releasing one of the most potent skin healers out there. Yes, it's goopy. Yes, it's kinda sticky. But it works. I smeared it on my son's cheeks before he went to bed, and by morning his skin looked healthier than ever. Naturally, I tried it on my own skin and found it worked just as great for me! (A word of caution: Unless you want to appear to be in a constant sweat, don't put this on during the day. It's rather shiny.)

Once again, this is a money saving tip, too. A bottle of vitamin E (go for the natural, not synthetic) is much cheaper than an eczema prescription or, heaven help us, those pricey night serum capsules for mom.

Calendula Oil

Take about a cup of the dried calendula flowers and place them in a clean glass jar that has a tight-fitting lid. Cover the flowers with a good fresh olive oil, and let the mixture sit for one to two weeks. Every day flip the jar upside down and back to help mix it. I like to let my jar sit in a sunny window so the sun can help the fusion process. (Just don't let it get too hot.) After a week or two, strain the oil through some cheesecloth or a strainer into another clean jar. You can rub this oil right on the eczema or put some in his bath water. The oil can be used for diaper rash, too. It's good for adult dry skin, as well, and this one jar should last your family a long time.

Aloe Vera Gel

While you're waiting for that oil to be ready, you can try a pure aloe gel. Read the ingredients, though; some of them have alcohol, of all things, which could sting and further dry the skin. Or some oatmeal in the bath can be soothing. I haven't found these remedies to be a long-term solution like the calendula oil or vitamin E, but they can provide some comfort until your oil is ready for use.

Fevers

If baby has a fever, remember this first: Fevers are nature's way of fighting off infection and illness, and are not always a reason for concern. Sometimes it's okay to treat it yourself and wait it out. There are times, however, when a fever warrants a visit with your pediatrician. We'll cover that here, along with some handy fever lowering remedies.

Vaccine Induced Fevers

One of the worst parts of getting babies vaccinated is the knowing, or not knowing, what is to follow. Will there be crying? Sleeplessness? Crankiness? And those are just your own side effects. What about baby? Many babies end up feeling like they have a touch of the flu, and it's not uncommon for a baby to run a slight fever. There's one natural remedy that can help ease a baby's fever after vaccinations. Just a couple drops of peppermint or chamomile essential oil in a bath is not only soothing to the discomfort after those shots, but it can get baby through that feverish part a little quicker.

If you're like me and you obsess over the side effects and toxins that are sometimes present in vaccines, there is a homeopathic remedy that can be used called thuja. Get the tablets at 6x strength and administer those two times daily for two to three weeks after the injections. It is said these tablets help remove the excess toxins from the body. A good health food store should be able to point you toward the correct tablets. Remember, homeopathic tablets just melt under the tongue, so it's nice and easy for little ones. They're usually sweet tasting, too, so they won't mind the inconvenience.

Ask your doctor what side effects to expect from any vaccines you choose to do, and which side effects are serious enough to come back into the office. When babies and young children get their vaccines, they'll sometimes feel achy and feverish for up to 24 hours. This might come across as crabbiness, tiredness, or fussiness. So be extra patient, give lots of cuddles, and plenty of kisses until it's all over. But if anything about your baby's behavior raises those parental alarm bells, call your doctor, no matter how silly the concern might seem to you.

The Bath

Try a warm bath, rather than cool, to bring down that fever. The warm water is actually safer, as cool water can reduce the fever too quickly. Allow your baby to sit in the tub until the water starts to cool, and then towel him off thoroughly.

Wiping Down

Using warm water, wet a washcloth and wipe down your baby gently. Not only will this ease the fever, the gentle interaction can soothe some fussiness. For extra calming power, use a warm, mild chamomile tea instead of plain water.

Fluid Intake

Make sure your baby is getting plenty of fluids. Offer formula or breast milk more often than usual; also make sure to offer water in a bottle for babies six months and up. Just make sure the water doesn't replace regular mealtimes.

What's Normal?

So what's a normal temperature and what's not? Here's a handy list you can copy and hang in your medicine cabinet:

Normal: 97 - 99°F (36 - 37.2°C)
Low-Grade: 99 - 100.9°F (37.3 - 38.3°C)
Common Fever: 101 - 103.5°F (38.4 - 39.7°C)
High Fever: Over 103.6°F (over 39.8°C)
Infants: Any fever warrants a doctor's visit.

Babies three to six months: See a doctor if fever over 101°F.

Babies six months and older: See a doctor if fever over 103°F.

Instincts Above All!

Most importantly: Follow your gut instincts, moms and dads. If something just plain doesn't feel right, call your pediatrician immediately.

SIDS

In the early 1990s, New Zealand had the highest infant mortality rate related to SIDS. More than two per 1,000 babies were dying of this horrible syndrome until a New Zealand scientist and chemist named Dr. Jim Sprott made an earth-shattering discovery: Crib mattresses treated with fire retardants were producing highly toxic nerve gases. Dr. Sprott realized baby fluids were seeping into these mattresses and creating a common fungus often found in mattresses. This fungus produces a heavier-than-air poisonous gas which hovers just at the surface of the mattress.

This fits much of what we do know of SIDS: Laying a baby on his back reduces the risk. If he's on his back, his mouth and nose are a little further from the gases. A family's second baby is more susceptible than a first, a third child more susceptible than a second, and so on, because it's common to reuse a baby mattress for the infancy of several children within a family. And babies of single parents have an even higher risk of SIDS. Often living on a tighter budget, it is much more common for single parents to resort to a previously used mattress, thus increasing the risk. Since we know used mattresses present a higher risk, it stands to reason that the more babies who have slept on a mattress, the more possibility these gases exist.

In 1994, Dr. Sprott created a mattress wrap that blocks these gases. The information was publicized through New Zealand, and since then, of the over 100,000 babies to sleep on this wrap, not one has died of SIDS. Not one.

In 2002, German doctor Hannes Kapuste published statistical results of the New Zealand mattress wrapping campaign. He stated: "...the statistical proof that mattress-wrapping prevents cot death (SIDS, crib death) is 1018 i.e. one billion billion times the level of proof which medical researchers generally regard as constituting certain proof of a scientific proposition."

In October of 2008, the news hit the fan here in the U.S.: It was now scientifically proven that if you put a bedroom fan in your baby's room, you could reduce the risk of SIDS by up to 72%. But did this story break in the UK? In Australia, New Zealand, the rest of the civilized world? Nope. Not news there. Why? Because in the rest of the civilized world, flame retardant chemicals in baby mattresses are viewed as the cold hard cause of SIDS. It has been scientifically researched over and over in Europe, Australia, and New Zealand. The results are always the same: When a newborn baby wets a mattress, the moisture is trapped inside. The mixture of urine and the flame retardant chemicals (banned in the aforementioned countries and continents) causes a chemical reaction, leading to a gas which floats up to breathing level for newborns. That's why the fan works; it blows away the gases. The media here in the U.S. stated the "prevailing theory" on SIDS was that infants were re-breathing carbon dioxide and didn't have the strength to move away for fresh air. "For whatever reason," one article stated, the carbon dioxide became trapped within the baby's lungs and caused death. (You can read that article here.) If that is the case, why would the risk increase for every following baby within a family? Does the second born have smaller airways, the third born smaller yet? Absolutely not.

When I first learned that SIDS could be prevented if I protected my son from his mattress (you can't buy mattresses without these dangerous fire retardants in the U.S. unless you purchase one of just a few safe but pricey mattresses), I came across Dr. Sprott's mattress cover. This was in 2006, but the covers are still available worldwide and the price is still unbeatable. For around 40 U.S. dollars (shipping from New Zealand included), you can purchase a food grade BPA-free impermeable plastic cover that is sort of like sticking your baby's mattress inside a giant freezer bag. The bag has no smell and no outgassing, and none of the phosphorus. It's easy to clean, so if there are any diaper overflows, it'll be even easier to sanitize than the mattress's original surface. If your baby sleeps in your bed, there are co-sleeper/playpen sizes too.

In case you're wondering, I get no kickbacks from Dr. Sprott, and I have absolutely no affiliation. I'm sure the people at Cot Life 2000 don't even know I exist. I'm just a happy, grateful customer that wants to help spread the word about SIDS prevention.

To read more about the research behind SIDS and to purchase a mattress cover, visit Stop SIDS Now.

Sleep Solutions

Days with a new baby are filled with love and wonder; but they're also filled with hard work and exhaustion! Sometimes the best thing for everybody is a good night's sleep. What do you do if your baby doesn't agree with this idea? Here are a few helpful tricks.

Baby Genius Harvey Karp

That same good doctor who advised me on breastfeeding also told me to get a copy of Harvey Karp's book, The Happiest Baby on the Block. What I learned about coercing my baby to go to sleep I used throughout my child's babyhood. Karp encourages what he calls the 5 S's. In a nutshell, the 5 S's are: Swaddling, Side or Stomach (not for sleep but for soothing), Shush, Swing, and Suck.

I learned to swaddle right away, and while it took several frustrating tries to get it right, I eventually became a swaddling expert. Nothing comforts a newborn like wrapping him properly so he feels safe and secure!

Side or stomach teaches that a newborn is more comfortable in these positions; and while you don't want to lay a baby on her stomach or side for bedtime, it's often helpful for calming the baby to hold her so she's either facing down or on her side. Once she's calm, you can lay her on her back for sleep.

Shushing is pretty much what it sounds like: While holding your swaddled baby on her side or her belly, make the "Shhhh!" sound loudly in her ear. Newborns aren't used to silence; they've just spent nine months in a very noisy place, listening to swooshing, gurgling, bubbling, and everything you said and did. Silence can be scary!

Swinging is the next component and can be added while doing all the others. A gentle jiggling of the baby is often comforting. Just be certain you don't shake. Instead, the movement should be more like shivering, just enough to move the baby no more than an inch back and forth.

Finally, sucking is added to the routine. A pacifier or a thumb works well for many babies, giving them comfort.

If you're still waiting for the arrival of your baby, be sure to add Harvey Karp's book to your baby shower wish list. While this gives you a rundown and can help if you need the information now, the book is filled with helpful information to aid new parents.

Make a Bedtime Ritual

Establishing a bedtime ritual can be key to helping your baby go to sleep. Start it each evening at the same time, and keep things quiet for your baby and keep the lights low while you prepare. These are the same cues all of our bodies rely on for a good night's sleep, but with our modern lifestyles, we've forgotten them. For a baby they're especially important.

As you get baby all cleaned up and in his jammies, you can hum quiet tunes, rub on some soothing natural lotion or salve, and perhaps throw in a little foot massage. Once baby is prepped for bed, make sure the room is dark and peaceful. Turn on a humidifier, both for the important added humidity and for the soothing sounds. Eventually, your baby will experience all of these things and begin to feel sleepy. By the time the nighttime feeding comes around, he'll be more than happy to hit the hay.

A Little Night Music

A mobile or musical lullaby toy often works wonders too, don't forget. My son had an under-the-sea toy that he could turn on himself by pushing the fish. As soon as he was old enough to work it, he could reach his little foot up and give the button a push. There were many nights I heard the soft music coming from his room at two or three in the morning, and I was grateful I didn't have to help him fall back asleep!

If your baby is especially stubborn about bedtime, you might try putting a small CD player or mp3 player in the corner of the room. Go for lullabies, soothing classical music, ocean or womb sounds, or bedtime music made especially for babies. And if you've ever noticed a specific sound tends to lull your baby to sleep (like the vacuum cleaner or the clothes dryer), you can even record the sound yourself and make your very own "mixed tape" for baby. Or if you have an external speaker for your smartphone, there are numerous free apps out there that feature relaxing sounds, including heartbeats and womb ambience.

Crying It Out

I have to admit that, while I have heard of people who said allowing their baby to cry it out worked for them, I never had the stamina for it. I tended to wait a bit to see if he'd sort things out on his own and go back to sleep. Sometimes he did, and sometimes he didn't. While my son started out as an excellent sleeper, he didn't stay that way. We hit a period that, while it only lasted a couple of months, felt like an eternity. Night after night, nap after nap, I struggled to get my son to sleep. We attempted to let him cry it out, but I melted within a few minutes. It felt horrible. What did seem to work was keeping music in his room; and while I refused to sleep next to his crib (I knew mothers who did that and never got to stay up past dark again), I did start reading near him until he drifted off. It didn't last forever, he felt secure, and we all got some sleep.

A dear friend of mine, Ann, has raised five babies so she knows a thing or two about getting them to sleep. Like me, she doesn't have the steely stomach for crying it out. Instead, she reassures the baby by entering the room, putting a hand on baby's back, and saying, "I love you and I'll see you in the morning." Not through gritted teeth or frustration, but with as much love as she can muster. She repeats this every ten minutes until the baby has quieted. She says it took each of her babies about two nights of this routine before they got the hint.

Wish I'd known her when my son was going through his "Late Night with Baby" stage!

Whether or not you choose the "crying it out" method is ultimately up to you. Every baby is different; after all, they're only human. But for me, I tend to agree with author of the book Secrets of the Baby Whisperer by Tracy Hogg, RN, who feels it's in the baby's best interest to go into the room whenever she cries, hold her a moment, then put her back to bed — no matter how many frustrating times that may occur.

Naps Are Essential

I've met too many parents who give up on naps early in their baby's life because the baby "just doesn't want to." Instead, they have a cranky baby who, by nighttime, is so exhausted he couldn't sleep even if he wanted to. They try everything, and eventually allow their tiny infant to stay up until they go to bed themselves, often at ten or eleven at night, because "our baby doesn't need much sleep." Of course he does! He needs much more than we adults do. No matter how frustrating it is on a parent's end, the baby has to get naps in, or at least what resembles a nap. Consistency helps. When your baby is able to get naps during the day, they're able to sleep better at night. It sounds counterintuitive, but it works.

Peaceful Days

Experts say that peaceful days for baby lead to better sleep patterns at night. Laying around all day shaking a rattle might not seem like stressful work, but babies pick up on everything around them. Everything is new, everything has to be mentally processed; every sound, sight, smell. Every new visitor who looks over the edge of a bassinet and squeals. Every trip to the brightly lit grocery store and the noisy car wash. It all adds up. Babies can get stressed, too; this also means if there is stress in your household such as fighting, chaos, noise, etc., baby can pick up on that and have a hard time getting to sleep at night. While we can't make everything perfect (life isn't, after all), doing your best to make sure the home is a peaceful, loving place will allow your baby to transition from a lovely day into a quiet bedtime and a restful sleep. She's gonna need it if she's got more visitors scheduled for tomorrow!

A Good Night's Sleep for All! (This Means You)

I remember a time writing an entry in my blog dkMommySpot.com on baby food combinations. After I'd published it, I went back through some previous entries to look something up. Lo and behold, only two weeks before, I'd written an article on the same exact topic — different food combinations, but the article was basically the same thing. When I read over the first article, I barely remembered writing it. Why? Sleep deprivation.

Parents of babies very rarely escape being denied a full eight hours of sleep. Some parents can't get a full night's sleep even up to baby's second year, and I've met frustrated moms and dads who have struggled into older years too. So what do we do, sleepy moms and dads? Hang up our sleeping caps until Junior graduates Harvard? Possibly so. But at least there are a few tips to get us through the first stages of babyhood.

Sleep When Baby Sleeps

A load of diaper doo, right? We've all heard that old chestnut, and if you're a working mom, it may be virtually impossible. But it can at least be done on the weekends. Saturdays are a great time to nap in shifts. Take turns with your spouse and one at a time, hole up in the bedroom with earplugs and without the (gasp!) baby monitor. Let the other parent sit with the kids while you get some much needed rest. When you're done, switch off. Now everyone's rested, at least for an afternoon.

A Cozy Corner

If you're up a lot with your baby in the wee hours, make sure you've got a comfortable setup. I still miss that little corner of my son's nursery. I had an antique rocking chair with an upholstered seat, a Boppy pillow to help with nursing, a foot stool, a side table with some books, a lamp on a dimmer switch, and a glass of water. If my son woke up in the night and I had to nurse him, I at least had comfortable surroundings. I still didn't get any sleep, but I was well read, and since I kept comfortable, it was easier for me to doze back off once I got back to bed.

Chamomile Once Again

If you breastfeed, drink some chamomile tea about an hour before your baby's last feeding before bedtime. You'll calm down, and the effects of the tea will pass to your baby, aiding in a deeper sleep for her.

There's no magic solution to getting a full night's sleep when baby doesn't want to, but at least there are some creative ideas out there to try. In the meantime, think of all the great stories you're saving up. You can tell people how you diapered the wrong end or how you (did I do that?) burned a pot of beans that stunk up the neighborhood when you had to set the smoking heap outside to cool off. And when your little one grows up, has a baby, and becomes sleep deprived, you can finally have a nice laugh. And some sleep.

Teething

Teething typically begins somewhere around the fifth or sixth month, but some babies show symptoms as early as the fourth month. If your baby is acting unusually irritable, if there's heavy drooling, biting on everything she can get a hold of, or a fever under 100°F, or if she's wakeful or restless, she may be experiencing teething. Other symptoms that are common would be facial rashes (sometimes more concentrated on the chin from all that drooling), red and swollen gums, or hardened gums.

Note: Babies who run a fever over 100°F and have diarrhea should be seen by a doctor, as these symptoms may not be related to teething.

The Usual Remedies

The most common things parents reach for when teething becomes a pain are teething gels and teething rings. But are they the best solutions? These days many doctors agree that teething gels hinder baby's ability to swallow, possibly causing choking. And the typical teething ring has had its own controversy surrounding the materials it's usually made of, namely the things that make the plastic pliable, such as BPA. So what's a health-conscious parent to do?

If you're going for a teething toy, make sure that any liquid-filled toy you purchase is filled with nothing more than water. These can be refrigerated but not frozen. Also make sure it's a safe BPA-free plastic. One sure way is to give it a whiff. If you smell a strong odor, there's a good chance that toy contains those chemicals you want to steer clear of. BPA-free toys are often marked as such.

Homeopathic Teething Tablets

Homeopathic tablets were a lifesaver for my son. When he started teething, he went from a pleasant baby who very rarely shed a tear to a weeping, noisy fountain. I was at a loss as to how to help him. When I discovered homeopathic teething tablets, I thought I'd give them a whirl; they're safe, natural, and baby can't overdose. (Still, follow the indications carefully.)

Homeopathic tablets are easily administered to babies of any age. They dissolve quickly, so all you have to do is put the recommended dosage under the tongue and hold your finger in the baby's mouth until the tablets dissolve. Teething tablets generally ease the discomfort and restlessness, but don't fear — they won't dope up the baby. The restfulness to follow is usually a result of relief from pain.

For those of you who are skeptical of the whole homeopathic thing, let me just say this: I used to be too. But my baby had no idea what a homeopathic tablet was or what it might do for him. No power of suggestion here. All I knew was that my baby stopped crying after he'd had his tablets. That was enough to convince me there was something to homeopathic remedies, after all. I've since used them for other things, and I still get surprised at the results.

Herbs

While not all herbs are safe for babies just because they're safe for you, there are some that you can try. This is where we'll revisit chamomile.

Chamomile can be given as a tea to ease the restlessness of teething. If you're breastfeeding, you can drink the tea yourself, which is a great way to calm you both down after an afternoon of crying. It only takes about 15 to 30 minutes for what you eat and drink to reach the breast milk, where it stays and reaches its peak in two to six hours. Or if you prefer, you can give chamomile tea in a bottle to your baby. To prepare for a bottle, use ½ teaspoon chamomile to a cup of almost boiling water. Steep the tea for five minutes and strain it thoroughly. Make sure it's a safe temperature, same as you would for milk or formula. Test a small amount on the inside of baby's arm first, just to make sure he's not one of the very few allergic to chamomile. If no reaction occurs after several hours, you can give this to your baby up to three times a day. Although as much as five ounces can be given at any one time, beware that chamomile can have a constipating effect. Also beware that any tea is a diuretic. So if the point of the chamomile is to help baby sleep, giving too much may wake him up sooner than you'd like with a wet diaper.

One last way for baby to enjoy the benefits of chamomile is to dip a clean washcloth in some chilled tea. Let him chew on it, or you can gently rub it on his gums. The chamomile has an antiseptic property, and it's important to keep those gums healthy, especially during teething. My dentist told me that keeping my son's gums clean with a damp washcloth during teething would actually lessen the discomfort, as the bacteria in the mouth only aggravates teething pain.

Eat Your Fruits & Vegetables, Dear!

What you feed your baby at this tender young age very much influences what he'll turn to later in life. It's why pediatricians encourage introducing a variety of foods when baby is learning to eat solids. It's also a reason this next tip is such a great one, serving a few purposes at once.

For a fun and soothing teething treat, try giving baby a cleaned piece of organic fruit or vegetable, chilled or frozen first. Perfect for noshing on would be the fatter half of an organic carrot or a nice chunk of cooled celery. Keep a dish in the refrigerator with a few of these on hand. That way, when your baby starts to yelp about the pain of teething, you have a chilled chewy at the ready. My son loved his carrot and celery sticks most of all. When he was about eight or nine months of age, he'd get upset if we needed to take them away. (Make sure you watch closely. When teeth start to emerge, baby may be able to start biting off small chunks.

Always supervise.)

If you'd like to try some of the smaller or mushier fruits and vegetables, get a piece of unbleached cheesecloth and cut out a square. Cheesecloth works well because it's free of lint, it's cheap, and it's disposable. If you can't find it at your local store, try online. Many online health food stores sell it for a reasonable price, and it can be had on Amazon in an array of prices. Put something like frozen peas, frozen banana, or frozen grapes in the middle of the fabric and tie it in a secure, tight knot. This is an excellent way for baby to get tastes for new foods too, and they feel pretty independent feeding themselves. But as always, keep a close eye on him to make sure he doesn't open the cloth.

Teething can be painful and challenging for parent and child both, but having a few tricks ready to go can help get everyone through it a little easier. Being prepared is a definite way of giving you peace of mind when the time comes. When a bout of teething is done, everyone is congratulated with a new toothy grin. What could be better than that?

Why Organic?

I know what you're thinking: It's more expensive. It's hard to find. Sometimes it looks funny, and there's usually real dirt on it. We're talking organic produce; but there's more to it than slightly smaller apples, and potatoes shaped like Richard Nixon. So what's the deal with organic produce, anyway?

Anything certified as organic needs to be produced without the use of antibiotics, synthetic hormones, and genetic engineering. That's scientific mumbo jumbo for "it's real." Organic fruits and vegetables are more nutrient rich, as well. For instance, studies show that organic broccoli contains more calcium and magnesium than broccoli that is not organic.

A fantastic reason to go organic is the avoidance of insecticides. Feeding your children organic food protects them from these chemicals, some of which are linked to the disruption of neurological development in infants and children.

One of my favorite reasons for going organic: It tastes so good! Organic fruits and vegetables often have a much better flavor. Personally, I find the carrots so much tastier, the bananas sweeter, the apples more flavorful. We eat as much organic produce in our home as we can, and it makes me feel good. Because I know I'm offering my son the best of the best — the safest, healthiest, tastiest way to enjoy fruits and vegetables. So grab that shopping basket. Who knows? You may just find an organic pomegranate shaped like Lyle Lovett.

The Question of Soy

Perhaps you've heard that soy is a big no-no for babies and young children; and for everyone else, for that matter. I've heard it all too, enough to start a research fest in which I looked to the opinions and hard facts from numerous doctors and nutritional experts that I trust and respect. I also looked for new information from people I didn't know so well.

A cursory look on Google made it abundantly clear: The overwhelming opinion on the matter is that soy is not only bad for your baby but downright dangerous. According to a scan down the search results, it's as if soy is the root of all health evils. Initially, I was alarmed. So I began to dig. As I researched several claims on blogs, articles, and websites, I was led back to the same root source time and time again: the Weston A. Price Foundation. Their site seemed to have everything laid out there for me, no questions needed. But they also advise a diet high in saturated fats, even for infants. Their homemade baby formula recipes suggest combining ingredients such as butter, olive oil, cow's cream, even liver. For newborns.

Other advice offered is that eating poached brains is healthy indeed and should be consumed regularly, and readers are advised to hide it in their family's food if they're opposed to brains (despite things such as Mad Cow Disease). Butter and butter fat are considered "super foods." And it is recommended that raw vegetables are usually unhealthy and should instead be sautéed in butter before serving. This is all based on the ideas of a dentist, Weston A. Price, who did a lot of important research — in the 1930s.

While my intention isn't to break out into a diatribe against the Winston A. Price Foundation, I felt it was worthy of touching on since this seems to be the source of all the anti-soy hype. What's in soy that's got them so worked up? Isoflavones (otherwise known as phytoestrogen, a plant estrogen). Interestingly, isoflavones are also found in garlic, flax seeds, sesame seeds, peanuts and many other foods that aren't up for debate.

On the flip side of the coin are people who have done their research in abundance, people such as Dr. Joel Fuhrman who advocates a diet high in nutrient dense greens, vegetables, and fruit. (He isn't anti-meat, mind you; but he is for healthy moderation.) Dr. Fuhrman states that, while processed soy products such as the isolated soy in protein powders is unhealthy, whole unprocessed soy products such as tofu, edamame, and tempeh provide meaningful health benefits

Dr. Andrew Weil said, "There is no scientific data suggesting that soy consumption leads to mineral deficiency in humans." In response to the question "Can soy feminize a boy?" he stated that, "When you consider that millions of men in China, Japan, and other Asian countries have had soy foods in their daily diets from earliest childhood, you can appreciate that the plant estrogens they contain have no discernible effect on male sexual development, and no feminizing effects at all. Given the huge populations of Asian countries there's no reason to think that soy affects male fertility, either."

While we're checking in on what some of our favorite nutrition-loving doctors are saying, let's get Dr. Oz's take. He stated that, "...Asians who typically eat a diet rich in soy products, fish, and fiber are known to have lower rates of breast cancer, high blood pressure, and heart disease. Yet when they move and adopt a westernized diet stacked with meat and processed foods, their health profile is negatively impacted. This suggests that the health they enjoyed at home may not be due to genetics alone, but their diet as well." Dr. Oz recommends that, like the Asians, Americans should focus on a balanced amount of soy, which would be about one serving a day; Dr. Weil recommends two servings. Either way, this is less than the daily average soy intake of the average Asian. Dr. Oz also warns to stay away from "frankensoy" products. Stick with the unprocessed.

So where does that leave baby in regards to soy formulas, which contain processed soy? This is a question you'll have to discuss thoroughly with a trusted pediatrician who understands your desire to keep things natural, before you make final formula decisions. The American Academy of Pediatrics, however, recommends cow's milk based formulas over soy, as cow's milk is closer to human breast milk than processed soy. Dr. Fuhrman says there are, indeed, legitimate claims over the health concerns of soy based infant formulas, as soy formulas tend to have a higher content of aluminum than that of cow's milk formulas. Again, we're talking processed soy. An edamame bean, on the other hand, is not in danger of giving you a dose of aluminum.

Keeping this all in mind, some of my baby food recipes contain whole soy products like soy milk, edamame, and tempeh. I highly recommend you always search for organic, GMO-free soy in order to gain the best possible benefits. Don't rely on soy as an everyday staple, just like you shouldn't rely on rice cereal or teething biscuits or bananas as being a constant go-to food. The key is always variety, in every aspect of nutrition.

Proper Baby Nutrition

If you decide to make your own baby food, the chance to offer your baby many different tastes and textures is endless. In fact, the greater the variety you offer to your little one, the more adventurous her tastes will be when she becomes old enough to choose on her own. She'll also tend to gravitate to those foods she ate even in her earliest days of solid foods. That's why it's so important to try a wide variety with your baby. But it's easy to get into a feeding rut when we're such busy parents. From my own experience, I loved banana day because it was so easy — just mash that thing up with a fork, maybe add a splash of water to get the right consistency, and you're all set. No cooking, no waiting for food to cool. No defrosting. How nice it would have been to feed my son bananas every day! But of course that's not the making of a well-balanced diet. Unless you happen to be raising a chimpanzee.

So how do we manage to provide that well-balanced diet? And what if our baby's discerning palate spits out half the menu? When my son was experimenting with solids, I introduced broccoli into his diet. Did he like it? Decidedly not. But mixed with applesauce, he tried to rip the bowl out of my hand and ate as fast as I could shovel it. Sometimes the trick is in the combinations. Cheating? Not really. After all, your baby is still eating the "dreaded" fruit or vegetable; the nutrients are going in and so is the taste, albeit much disguised. Eventually, they may learn to like it without the clever cover-up.

With a little creativity, we can keep those different foods coming. It's so important at this stage. We're literally setting up the food map in their heads as to how they eat later in life. If we're clever and we keep at it without giving up, we're giving our children a great gift of health. They'll grow to view fruit as a treat and not something in the lunch box to trade for a

Twinkie. They might even eat their spinach.

Getting the Right Nutrients

Your baby's brain will continue to grow and develop until he's in his teens, so it's important to feed that growing mind with healthy brain food. Omega-3 fatty acids are an essential building block for your baby and can actually boost his IQ, so it's important to find ways to incorporate foods into your child's diet that are rich in omega-3s. Children with a low intake of DHA, a certain type of omega-3, can suffer from things like ADHD, sleep problems, aggressiveness, depression, dyslexia, impulsiveness, temper tantrums, and even manic depression. But the good news is, there are ways to make sure our children aren't lacking in this all-important fatty acid.

If your baby is breastfed, you'll be supplying lots of DHA. As a nursing mother, you can take omega-3 supplements yourself. (You can find those that are derived from the oil of mercury-free fish, but some supplements are made from plant algae instead.) Some baby formulas include this element, but if you're using one without it, look for one that supplies DHA or ask your pediatrician for a supplement.

If your baby is eating solids, you can feed him plenty of green vegetables to ensure he's getting his omega-3s. Young children and nursing moms can get more omega-3s through walnuts and flax seed too. (When you use flax, make sure it's ground first. The outer hull is hard and doesn't digest well. We run our flax through a coffee grinder before adding a couple teaspoons to smoothies or sprinkled on cereal.)

One of my biggest concerns in starting my son's life on a mostly vegan diet was, "Where would he get the right balance of vitamins and minerals?" Calcium and protein were two things I wanted to be sure of, considering my son started his first few years mostly vegetarian. I grew up eating a standard American diet with plenty of dairy products and meat, so it was hard sometimes for my mind to shift gears. Like most Americans, I had no idea calcium and protein were found in fresh fruits and vegetables. In fact, if you tell most people they can get almost all the calcium and protein they need just from eating the right veggies, they'll probably think you're kidding. After I ran a check at NutritionData.com, I was happy to see that with the variety my son received each day, he met his needs in the calcium and protein departments, as well as other important vitamins and minerals. Running your own check by testing the foods you feed your baby regularly will give you a better idea of what she's getting and of what she needs.

Talk to Your Pediatrician First

Before introducing solid foods to your baby, make sure to get your pediatrician's input on the whens and the whats. Discuss possible food allergies for your baby, too. What I've put together for this book is meant only as a guide and not the end-all be-all on baby food and nutrition.

Baby Food by Age

One thing that confused me as a new mother, more than many aspects of raising a baby, was what to feed him and when. It was so exciting to start on solid foods, and it felt like a big step. But when you're making your own, you aren't depending on the store shelves telling you what your six-month-old is ready for. Sure, I could scan the shelves myself to see what the baby food producers were selling for babies my son's age. But half the fun in making my own baby food was having the freedom to introduce my baby to a wide variety of fruits and vegetables, right from the start.

One thing I wish I would have had in the beginning was a nice food chart, one that would outline age-appropriate foods and textures so I could be more at ease over the choices I was making. So here on the next several pages, you'll find a handy chart showing you just that:

foods right for you baby as the months progress, and how best to serve them. Keep in mind, this chart is general. Some babies don't tolerate certain foods as well as others. Also, always watch your baby closely when changing food textures to something chunkier than what they're used to. If it doesn't seem to be working, or you're simply uncomfortable with it, take a step back regardless of the age listed on the charts. You'll know when your baby is able to tolerate a little more heft in his fruit cup and when pureed is necessary. So don't sweat it. The important thing is for both you and your baby to have fun trying new foods. Bon Appétit, Baby!

When to Start

Most pediatricians agree that solid food shouldn't start until baby's sixth month, but in certain instances, a few will recommend starting solids as early as four months. Check with your pediatrician to find out when your baby should begin solids. After introducing a new food, make sure to offer that same food for three or four days before moving onto the next one. This will give you the chance to monitor for any side effects. Also keep an eye on baby's diaper "output" for any changes there.

Six to Eight Months

In the six- to eight-month range, food should be steamed or boiled, then pureed to a very smooth consistency. Strain out anything the least bit chunky. Your baby's first experiences with food should be smooth and easy to swallow. You can use a blender or a food processor; high powered blenders work especially well.

Grains: Rice, oatmeal, or barley cereals mixed with formula or breast milk.

Fruit: Bananas (pureed; the only one that you don't need to cook), pears, apples, apricots, peaches, nectarines, plums, and prunes.

Vegetables: Avocados, pumpkin, carrots, peas, yellow squash, zucchini.

Eight to Ten Months

Pureed and mashed foods work well for this age range, and by eight months fruit can be eaten raw. At about the nine-month period, introduce a slightly lumpier consistency. Finger food can also be started now, in the form of cooked bite-sized vegetables and melt-in-mouth foods. Start them slowly and always watch to see what your baby can handle. Each baby is unique in what he or she can tolerate.

Grains: Wheat cereals, graham crackers without honey, no-salt multi-grain crackers, teething biscuits, wheat germ, wheat or multi-grain toast.

Fruit: Blueberries, cantaloupe, kiwi, mangoes, papaya; pear and apple juice.

Vegetables: Asparagus, broccoli, cauliflower, eggplant, mashed white potatoes, beans and legumes (like split peas and lentils).

Meat: Lean beef, pork.

Dairy: Cream cheese, cottage cheese, American, Colby, and light cheddar cheeses, yogurt.

Ten to Twelve Months

At this stage, table foods are entering the diet more often. The number of teeth your baby has will play a big part in what they can and cannot handle, so watch closely.

Grains: Pastas, hard bagels, rice cakes.

Fruit: Cherries, citrus, dates, grapes cut in quarters..

Vegetables: Artichokes, beets, corn, cucumbers, spinach, tomatoes

Meat: Fish (cod and haddock), poultry.

Dairy: Whole eggs (at 12 months of age), whole milk (also at 12 months of age, but see note below), stronger cheddars, Gouda, Monterrey Jack, Muenster, provolone.

And While We're Talking Dairy...

Whether you have chosen breastfeeding or formula, at some point you will ask the question "When can I give my baby cow's milk?" Most people begin their children on cow's milk at about a year of age. But there are some things to consider before making the leap to dairy.

Milk has this funny way of bonding with the iron in the body and preventing its absorption into the system. In fact, milk is the leading cause of iron-deficiency anemia in babies and young children. This is a big reason experts advise strongly against giving infants cow's milk at all. But when they're older? Let's take a quick look at your baby's digestion.

The digestive tract of a baby has little tiny gaps between the cells. These darling little gaps allow for important antibodies from mom's milk to be able to seep into the bloodstream. Sometime before your baby's second birthday, these spaces seal up, preparing junior for some more serious "big boy or girl" digestion. It's plain to see, with such a wonderful example of how the body develops, how babies are perfectly built to accept human milk. Oddly, baby cows are perfectly designed to accept cow's milk.

If your baby has reached one year of age and that's when you plan to wean, talk to your doctor about using soy milk, which is more easily digestible. You can even make your own soy milk to avoid all the added ingredients in most store brands. I used a Tribest Soyabella Soy Milk Maker for years. (If whoever borrowed that would like to return it now, I'd be most grateful.) If you plan to give baby some cow's milk eventually, waiting until two years of age may be the better route.

Milk Consumption Chart

Here's a handy chart that tells you how much breast milk or formula. Keep in mind these vary greatly depending on the baby.

4 to 5 months: 30 ounces

5 to 6 months: 35 ounces

6 to 7 months: 28 ounces

7 to 9 months: 24 ounces

9 to 12 months: 22 ounces

Spices

When your baby hits the eight-month mark, you can introduce a few spices to her food. Keep it to a sprinkle, and try one spice at a time rather than a mix. This is to ensure there is no stomach upset; and if there is, you know what to leave out next time. These are a few baby-safe herbs and spices you can try, along with a benefit or two of each.

    Vanilla (antioxidant)
    Pepper (relieves gas)
    Garlic Powder (antibiotic)
    Basil (antibacterial)
    Rosemary (relieves gas, respiratory relief)
    Coriander (relieves gas, stimulates appetite)
    Dill (hiccups, colic, digestive problems)
    Oregano (antibacterial, antifungal)
    Lemon Zest (antifungal)
    Ginger (good for tummy upsets)
    Cinnamon (tummy upsets, diarrhea,

antifungal, antibacterial)

Mint (aids in digestion, temporary respiratory relief)

Nutmeg (aids in sleep, pain reliever)

Anise (colic, mild expectorant)

Homemade Baby Food Recipes

If you're ready to prepare your own baby food but you don't know where to start, here are a few recipes to get you going.

From 6 Months

Pear Applesauce

Peel, core, and boil or steam one apple and one pear until very soft. Mash or mix in blender until smooth. (For older babies, leave a little chunky for texture.) Sprinkle with a touch of cinnamon if you prefer.

Fruity Quinoa

Take the above recipe and add it to some cooked quinoa. You can thin this mixture with some breast milk or formula, if you prefer.

Homemade Baby Cereal

Sure, you can purchase some rice cereal in a cardboard box down at the grocer's, but it's quick and easy to make your own. Just grind some uncooked organic brown rice or slow-cook oats in your blender or a spice or coffee grinder (designated for this purpose, please — no one wants a caffeinated baby) until it's pulverized. To prepare it, add two tablespoons of the cereal to one cup of boiling water and whisk until smooth. You can add a bit of breast milk or formula if you'd like to give it a creamier consistency.

More Oatmeal, Peas

For dinnertime oatmeal, combine your homemade baby oatmeal and some breast milk until it's at the desired smooth consistency. Steam some organic peas (frozen are fine) until they're soft. Puree them in a blender with a bit of water until it's smooth with no lumps. Stir them into the oatmeal. This is a nice way to introduce peas to your baby because the oatmeal will probably be a familiar flavor and texture already.

Pumpkin Yumpkin

This recipe takes a bit more time, but it's a wonderful way to introduce a fun food to you baby. And if you're looking for a nice holiday recipe to take to Grandma's, you've got one now!

Get a small pie pumpkin and cut it in half, right through the middle. (You can leave the stem on one half.) Remove seeds. Put about an inch of water in a glass casserole dish and place the pumpkin halves inside, cut side down. Bake at 350°F until you can easily pierce the skin with a fork. Allow pumpkin to cool, then scoop the insides into a food processor. Peel and core two apples. Chop, then steam or boil them until soft. Place them in the food processor with the pumpkin. Add a dash of cinnamon, then puree.

From 8 Months

Mango Banana Puree

Peel and chop one mango and one banana. Puree in a blender or food processor until smooth.

Chia Porridge

Chia seeds are loaded with protein, omega-3s, fiber, and antioxidants. While I myself eat a similar dish made of whole chia as a breakfast food, it's a good idea to grind the chia just before use for your baby. Chia seeds are slippery little buggers and could otherwise present a choking hazard, albeit a minor one. Mix two or three teaspoons of ground chia with some breast milk or formula and allow it to sit for a couple of minutes. If it's too thick, stir in more liquid. (This does continue to thicken, so you'll want to wait another minute or two until you get the right consistency.) To this, you can add mashed fruit or pureed steamed carrots, perhaps a dash of spice like cinnamon to the fruit or a hint of dried basil or dill to the carrots.

Banana Yogurt

Mash ½ a banana with a fork. Add ½ cup plain Greek yogurt and mix. Experiment with adding a bit of pureed fruit such as peaches or blueberries for some delicious variation. Note: Yogurt and cheese are okay at this age even though it's dairy, because the lactose is broken down.

Green Bean Mash-Up

Mash some white potatoes with a bit of breast milk or formula. Add pureed green beans and mashed steamed carrots for a bowl of veggie goodness. For babies nine months and older, you can add a bit of texture by finely chopping the green beans and/or carrots.

Goodness it's Tofu

Steam summer squash, zucchini, and broccoli. Puree it all in a blender, together with a chunk of tofu. Stir in a bit of brown rice cereal and some hot water until it reaches a smooth, even consistency. For a touch of sweetness, you can add a bit of steamed and pureed apple.

From 10 Months

Banana Oatmeal with Molasses

Black strap molasses is a lovely, healthy sweetener that contains iron, calcium, magnesium, potassium, copper, and manganese. (Look for the word "unsulfured" on the label. Sulfur is sometimes added, and it's best avoided.) Prepare oatmeal as usual; mash ½ a banana in the bottom of a bowl with a fork. Add the oatmeal and a small spoonful of blackstrap molasses. You can also add a bit of breast milk or formula to thin down the cereal. Caution: Use only a small amount of the molasses, as it has a laxative effect.

Veggies and Pasta Italiano

Using equal quantities steamed green

beans and carrots, grind in food processor or blender until you get the desired consistency. Prepare very small pasta, such as organic whole wheat or rice pastina, according to package directions. (Use slightly less than the quantities of green beans and carrots.) Drain pasta and mix vegetables and pasta together. Freeze if desired.

Baby's Lentil Stew

Mix together equal portions well-cooked lentils, small pieces steamed green beans, and small pieces steamed carrots. Add some steamed pureed peas until you have a stew-like consistency.

Dark Leafy Green Goodness

Take two to three shredded leaves of organic kale, minus the middle tough part, steamed or boiled until soft (retain a little cooking water) ½ cored organic apple, and some organic baby cereal, enough for desired consistency. Put the cooked kale and the apple into a high powered blender and blend until smooth, with a little of the reserved cooking liquid. This makes a mush. Add cereal until you get the desired consistency. The apple adds a sweet flavor, and the cereal is a recognizable texture for babies, so getting them to eat it is pretty easy.

Baby's First Ice Cream

This recipe will make enough for you, too, so you're welcome. It's a dessert I make for my family on a regular basis, and it beats the sugar and empty calories of real ice cream while offering the rich, creamy texture and a phenomenal flavor that will make it hard to believe it's healthy. You can add other fruits as well, such as a small handful of frozen blueberries. Or puree some raspberries and drizzle it on top. A decadent start to life.

2 frozen bananas (Peeled, wrapped in plastic wrap, and frozen for a couple of hours.)

¼ cup soy milk

¼ tsp. real vanilla extract

Throw it all in a high powered blender. If your blender isn't high powered, break up the bananas a bit first. Run the blender until it becomes the consistency of soft serve ice cream. (Note: To avoid giving baby the "brain freeze" we all remember from childhood, allow the ice cream to melt a bit first. Or add some extra milk so it's slightly soupy.)

Baby Food Variety - Creating Your Own Combinations

One thing I've noticed about making your own baby food is that it's easy to get stuck in a cooking rut. Your favorite store always carries organic frozen broccoli, it's a quick solution to boil the apples now that you can peel one in under 30 seconds, and steaming a bag of frozen peas is a snap. But the one thing you don't want to do is to get into a habit of offering your baby the same foods over and over.

It Bears Repeating

Babies and children generally need about 11 tries before they learn to like certain foods. Starting them early on a wide variety can make things much easier when you are the parent to a picky toddler who would otherwise rather see peas fly than to eat them. Besides, with variety comes health and an exposure to more vitamins and minerals.

Baby Stew

When my son was old enough to try it, I discovered he wasn't too hip on green beans. I wanted him to have it in his diet because it's so healthy. But he wasn't buying it. He did, however, adore his carrots. So I tried mixing ½ carrots to ½ green beans, steamed and smashed. (Make sure you have the right consistency for the proper age. My son was about eight months old at this point.) He liked that combination so much that he was flapping his arms between every bite. It was like me with a 5-pound tray of chocolate brownies. Jackpot! Green beans were in his diet to stay.

Get creative with your baby's diet. Take a look at the colors of the fruits and vegetables, and make sure you vary them. Orange gives lots of beta carotene, such as yams and carrots. Dark green often means iron and calcium. Whites tend to contain starches, like rice or potatoes.

Blending foods together is not only a great way to add some variation, it's also a nice way to sneak in some new foods that maybe baby isn't so hot about at first. For instance, the first time I tried to feed my son lentils, he kept spraying them all over the front of my shirt in protest. I wanted to get legumes into his diet, so I started mixing them with some diced carrots, then hiding that mixture in pureed green beans. Bingo! Lentils disappeared without a trace. And no scraping dried bits of legume off my glasses. In the meantime he was adjusting to them being there, so eventually I could back off on some of the other ingredients so he could learn that lentils weren't so scary.

I call that technique "making baby stew." It's kind of fun, and the possibilities are endless. When your baby is learning to deal with textures in food, and she's exercising those gums and new teeth on a few chunks, mixing the chunky stuff in with some pureed vegetable can make the changeover less dramatic. Not all babies take kindly to going from warm smooth mush to having to chew. So compromise by mixing the two together, and your baby may have an easier time accepting diced fruits and veggies.

Getting Unconventional

Another creative way to depart from the norm is to try mixing fruit and vegetables together. One great food for any baby over the age of six months is avocado and banana. I just felt you cringe. But one mashed avocado and ½ a mashed banana blended together has a nice refreshing flavor. Go ahead — I dare you. Stick your finger in the food and try it for yourself. Even if you're not a fan of avocado, this one might grab you. If not, try something a little safer like blending cooked apples and carrots or cooked apples and sweet potatoes.

Continue to look for new and interesting foods good for your baby's age at your grocery store or health food store. Making a habit of looking for something to shake things up is a much better idea than making a habit of serving the same few combinations. Babies don't get sick of routine foods like we do; on the contrary, they seem to revel in it. Bringing new and interesting food to the table today will give you an adventurous eater in the future.

Finger Food Ideas

As your baby gets ready to experiment with finger foods, the fun (and the mess) really begins! It's time to crank out some variety and enjoy watching your baby sample new textures and flavors. Some he'll like and some he'll probably throw at the dog, but time and patience will give him an opportunity to adjust and find new favorites.

How to Get Started With Finger Foods

The most important factor is keeping a very close eye on what your baby can handle. Most babies can try a few finger foods when they're eight or nine months old, about the time they start attempting to swipe the spoon out of your hand or pull food off your plate. Start by sitting baby in the high chair and offering a few small pieces of soft food on the tray before them.

Watch and make sure the sizes of cubed foods are not too big, and that the food is soft enough to chew on with those baby gums. It's a constant adjustment and plenty of trial and error to find the right combination of size and consistency because every baby is different. The crucial thing is to be present and watch closely.

Simple Singles

One yummy finger food is the sweet potato. You can cut them in cubes, or when she's ready, cut them in strips. Start with cubes about ½ inch square or smaller. Boil them until they're soft but not falling apart. Allow to cool before serving. (Test one yourself first because these can retain quite a bit of heat in the center.)

Of course pieces of cut banana and kiwi are easy because you don't have to cook them first. Bananas are great take-along snack, no packaging required! Cubed apples and pears can be boiled or steamed, but if the pear is soft enough, you can serve it raw.

Another handy finger food is the green bean. Boil them until they are soft but not falling apart. You can either cut them smaller or serve them whole, depending on your baby's capabilities. Other fun vegetables are steamed broccoli or cauliflower for little "trees." Make sure they're soft enough, including the "trunks."

My son always loved edamame. Purchase frozen organic edamame pods and steam them according to directions (usually just a couple of minutes.) Wait for them to cool, then pop them out of the pod. They're a beautiful bright green color, they're loaded with protein, and are a fun food to exercise pinching skills. They also travel well if a snack is needed on the go.

Pasta is another favorite. Choose shapes such as spirals that can be cut small enough to handle and to reduce the risk of choking. You can serve them with a few small pieces of soft cheese for a bit of Italian flair at dinner.

Holy Guacamole Pitas

I've made guacamole a lot in my house,

and when my son was small, it didn't take me long to realize how much he loved sampling our snack. He also loved whole wheat pita bread, so I would squish a little guacamole in small pieces of pita to make him his own tiny sandwiches. Fun finger food, and so healthy too. This travels well if you pack the pita separately and assemble it on the spot. Avocados have the good fats you need, omega-3s, and nearly twenty other essential vitamins, minerals, and phytonutrients. Babies can eat plain smashed avocado from an early age because it's easy to digest. And avocados aid in the growth and development of the central nervous system and the brain. My, what a smart food.

Here's my favorite way to prepare guacamole, which is great for the whole family. The added ingredients are also wonderful for growing toddlers.

2 Haas avocados (look for slightly soft ones with a reddish color to the skin)

1 or 2 finely chopped garlic cloves

2 to 3 Tbs. finely chopped onion (unless gas is a concern)

½ finely chopped tomato

juice of ½ lemon

fresh chopped cilantro (a powerful mercury remover, by the way) – about 1 to 2 Tbs.

sea salt to taste (optional)

To the adult's portion, you can add ½ finely chopped jalapeño.

Run a knife the long way around an avocado, then twist it. Pop out the pit, scoop out the green stuff, and smash. Add the rest of the ingredients and mix well. Take a small chunk of whole wheat pita and split it open to form a little pocket. Smear some guacamole inside and close it back up.

Freezing Baby Food

So you've got all that fresh organic produce, and you're ready to start cranking out the most wholesome, healthy meals possible for your little darling. But that big bag of peas isn't going to last forever, and if you make the whole thing now, baby will be eating mashed peas morning, noon, and night for three days. Not to despair. Freezing the food is easy and it cuts down on your work time later. All your friends popping open jars of the store-bought stuff just *think* they have it easier. Wait until they see your freezer full of baby food goodness. They'll be as green as that bag of peas over there.

Naturally, the first step is to make the food. Try and get organic if you can. Some big box stores carry frozen organic produce. It's okay to start with frozen even if you plan to cook it and freeze it up again. If you have access to fresh, even better. But we all know it's hard to find fresh organic peaches year round if you're in the frigid north. Fresh or frozen, steam the vegetables when possible. It retains the most nutrients. Fruit can be boiled, steamed, or in the case of bananas and kiwis, even just mashed (see food chart for age appropriateness of raw fruit).

For freezing, I prefer one- or two-cup glass containers by either Pyrex or Anchor Hocking. They're a nice little size, you can freeze them safely, and they stack well in the freezer. I also like the fact that once the food is defrosted, I can either set the glass dish in a pan of shallow hot water, or bring some water to a low boil in a pan and just set that dish in there to warm the food through. Some moms freeze their food in ice cube trays. The portions are smaller, and you can defrost just the right amount, but I prefer freezing in slightly larger quantities, then using it for a few meals.

Make sure you mark the containers so you don't forget what's in there; small sticky notes work well. Always put the month, date, and contents on your labels. If you're making batches of broccoli, peas, and beans, you'll never be able to tell them apart once they're all stacked together. Also, make sure you rotate your stock. Try and use up the older frozen food first. I would recommend not keeping it for more than a month. The fresher the better — even when it's frozen.

If you're blending foods together for new and interesting flavors, you can either freeze the vegetables separate, or premix them. It can be handy to freeze them separately so you can choose what you want to mix up later. It gives you a little more freedom for mixing and matching.

For older babies who need a little texture, try running your vegetables through the food processor or a high powered blender until you get the desired consistency before steaming or boiling. This works well for larger chunks for finger foods, as well.

Now you've got beautiful rows of baby food lined up in your freezer. There is a wide variety of choices at the ready; just take out lunch and dinner selections in the morning, so they're all thawed in time for baby's grand organic feast. Believe me, there's nothing more satisfying than feeding your baby fresh organic food you've made yourself.

Cleaning With Baby in Mind

Cleaning takes on a whole new perspective for the first-time mommy, especially if she's health conscious about the products she uses. When I was pregnant I was already an advocate of chemical-free living, but waiting for the birth of our son, I saw even more cleaning products in our home I wanted to replace.

One of the best parts about making your own cleansers is the price. The difference is unbelievable. They're easy to make, finding ingredients is often as simple as stepping into your kitchen, and if baby happens to get into the cupboards, there's a good chance it's harmless or nearly so.

(Keep them out of reach anyway. No matter how safe your cleaners seem to be, children can get rather creative with stuff that's not theirs.)

Basic Home Cleanser

Probably the most versatile of home cleansers is white vinegar. I could devote a whole book just to the many uses of this wonderful stuff. In my house, a spray bottle of vinegar and water is the all-purpose cleanser of choice. Great on glass, counter tops, mirrors, windows, linoleum, baby toys; the list is endless. It even kills germs and bacteria. For this mixture, I use one part water to one part vinegar. If you don't want your house smelling like salad dressing, add a few drops of sweet orange or lemon oil. I often combine grapefruit, lime, and tangerine oils for a fresh citrus scent and a boost of citrus cleaning power.

In the laundry, vinegar can be used in the rinse cycle as a bleach alternative, a fabric softener, and a static inhibitor. It also kills germs and bacteria, something ordinary laundry detergent does not do. In the kitchen, you can mix it with water in a large bowl and soak breast pump components and bottle caps and nipples. And in baby's room, it's a safe cleanser for removing germs from crib bars, the changing table, and other surfaces.

Furniture Polish

When I was pregnant, I went through that big cleaning spurt that happens when you're in the last trimester and hardly able to move. I was scrubbing every square inch of anything sitting still and half the things that didn't. (Ah, the poor dogs.) Any fumes wafting from cleansers became even more of a nuisance to me than before pregnancy. When it came to polishing all the wood in the baby's room, I didn't want to use any old spray-on furniture polish filled with pretend lemon and something that smelled a little too close to airplane fuel. After doing some digging, I found a nice recipe for furniture polish that sent me into whole new ecstasies of dirt purging. Here's what I use now:

¼ cup vinegar

2 Tbs. olive oil

3 or 4 drops of lemon or sweet orange oil

Put the ingredients together in a container with a lid and shake until it's well blended. Use it just as you would any commercial polish: Apply it with a dry cotton cloth and buff to shine. The vinegar in this solution is a nice cleansing agent, and the oils nourish the wood and leave a warm glow, as well as a fresh clean scent. By the time my son was old enough to pull himself up on everything, I was glad he didn't have to ingest any jet fuel-scented polish. I still love that polish. Martha Stewart, eat your heart out.

Wood Floor Cleanser

You know by now that I like tea. Herbal teas are fantastic for what ails you or just as a comfort. Green tea is a great antioxidant and disease preventative. But what if I told you not to drink your tea? Right now my tea advice to you is this: Dump it on the floor! That's right. A safe and natural way to clean your wood floors is with regular black tea. Tannic acid does wonders for wood. Again, this is a cheap, safe, and natural solution that allows you to rid your cupboards of one or two more cleanser bottles.

Here's what you do: Just boil a quart of water and steep one or two tea bags until the water cools to room temperature. Take out the tea bags and use a soft cloth to dip in the tea. Wring out the cloth well, then wipe down the floors. Replace the cloth once it gets dirty.

Not only will your floors be nice and clean, you'll also be gently covering some of those little imperfections and Hot Wheels scratches. Now when your two-year-old decides to lick the floor (simply for experimental purposes, mind you), you won't have to worry about the dirt — or the chemicals.

Carpet Stains

When my son was about two, he decided to draw on his white bedroom carpet. The white carpet and white painted walls, which went throughout our entire house, was not my idea but the brilliant decorating scheme of the childless couple who lived there before us.

Unfortunately, my son chose the hot pink crayon for his very long arching stripe across the middle of the floor. These were washable name-brand crayons. They did not wash.

I admit it, I panicked. I had a bottle of nasty chemical-laden spot remover that had managed to stay in the house despite all my chemical-free tricks. Why I grabbed that first instead of my usual stuff, I'll never know, but I attacked the stain with the smelly gel. And guess what? His room reeked of it for days. The cleaner turned the bright pink stripe into a wide smudge of rose pink.

The second thing I grabbed was my trusty old bottle of vinegar and water, which did remove the stain completely. No more pink, and I've learned my lesson. Sometimes life happens and no manner of natural remedy will remove a stain, but it's always good to try it first. So for your average nasty carpet stain, try a mixture of ⅓ white vinegar to ⅔ water. Spray bottles are best; adjusting the spray nozzle to a stream can really knock out a stain. If it's a tough one, try sprinkling a little baking soda on the area and blot. Allow the area to dry thoroughly before vacuuming. It may take a few applications, but it's worth it!

Other carpet cleaning tricks:

Gum: freeze with an ice cube, then break it off the carpet.

Paint, makeup, staining goopy stuff: Scrape off with a dull knife, then try the vinegar mixture above or blot on rubbing alcohol. (Always test your carpet first in an inconspicuous area.)

Fruit Juice: If you have a wet vac, you can try sucking up as much as possible before blotting the area with a damp paper towel. I've used the vinegar spray with good success on fruit juice. Or try ½ tsp. dish soap in a quart of water and blot the area.

Honestly, I've used a wide variety of natural remedies over the years I had that white carpet, but for spot cleaning the best I found was the vinegar solution. It removed muddy dog prints, crayon, blueberry juice, dog "products" (need I say more?), coffee, and wine. I still keep a spray bottle at the ready under every sink in the house.

Natural Air Fresheners

I love making my own air fresheners. They're safe and cheap, and you can change scents easily whenever your olfactory lobes get bored. Here are some fragrant room spray recipes for you to try. Although they all call for a little vodka, I use just distilled water when I make small quantities. I find it works well without the vodka as long as the water is distilled, and it's one less ingredient you have to purchase.

The recipe is basically the same for all scents; just alter the essential oils. Regardless of scent, you mix together the essential oil with ½ tsp. vodka in a 16-ounce spray bottle. Shake well, then add two cups of water and shake again.

Here are some essential oil combinations

to get you started. After that, it's all up to your imagination! And your nose...

Lavender-Citrus: 15 drops lavender oil, 10 drops grapefruit oil

Forest Freshness: 10 drops sandalwood oil, 10 drops pine oil, 10 drops juniper oil

Antiseptic Freshener: This one is great for a house that has been under siege by colds and flu: 20 drops juniper oil, 20 drops eucalyptus oil, 20 drops lavender oil.

Make sure not to use this spray on wood surfaces or fabric. I have sprayed mine on fabric numerous times, but for that I tend to use just a couple drops of oil in a small (maybe 2-ounce) spray bottle of water. One of my favorite uses on fabric is the dog bed. I use about five or six drops of cedarwood oil in a 2-ounce spray bottle of water and shake. Spray it on the cushion and around the area where the dog hangs out. It helps chase away any lurking fleas and freshens the doggie smell too.

Cleaning the Kitchen

If you want that kitchen sparkling but you don't want the cabinet under your sink to look like a mad scientist's laboratory, ditch those nasty bottles of harmful cleansers and replace them with these safe and, might I add, cheap items.

Smelly cutting board? Wet it down and rub a little dry mustard on it. Let it sit a couple minutes and rinse. To disinfect, I keep an old dish soap bottle handy with the ½ water, ½ white vinegar solution. I squirt some on the board, scrub, and rinse. (This is also a great cleanser for fruits and veggies instead of the costly Fit.)

Gas Stove Tops: For a great nonabrasive clean, remove your burners and sprinkle on some baking soda. Mist the stove top with your vinegar and water. With a damp cloth, scrub away the crud, rinse the cloth, and wipe away the baking soda. This is one of my favorite natural cleaning tips — it will outdo any of those expensive cleaners.

Dishwasher Odors: Sprinkle some borax in your dishwasher, particularly in the bottom. Leave it overnight and wipe it away in the morning with a damp cloth. Let the next load of dishes do the rest of the cleaning.

Cleaning the Bathroom

Chrome fixtures: To brighten and remove all that spotty stuff on your bathroom chrome, spray on straight white vinegar and wipe off with a clean dry cloth or sponge. I like to let the vinegar sit for a couple minutes first. You can also use lemon juice instead of vinegar. There's just something about a lemony smell that lets everyone know you've been working really hard and deserve to prop your feet up. Buff with a microfiber cloth for extra shine.

Removing hairspray buildup: Use a paste of baking soda and water to get rid of hairspray buildup on countertops and sink fixtures. You can also use equal parts rubbing alcohol and water, but of course rubbing alcohol is something you want well out of the reach of children.

Mineral deposits on the shower head: Put straight white vinegar in a plastic sandwich or freezer bag and tie it on the shower head overnight. In the morning, give the fixture a good scrub with a cleaning brush. The rubbery bristled type works well.

Toilet Bowl: Yes, vinegar can even be used to clean that toilet bowl. Dump a large bowl of water into the toilet bowl to get the water level down, pour the vinegar around the bowl, and scrub just as you would with any other toilet cleaner. You can also add a few drops of sweet orange oil to further disinfect.

Be sure to set a little bottle of your homemade natural air freshener in the bathroom, too.

Laundry

Nothing adds to the laundry pile like having a baby! All sorts of stains unique to these tiny bundles suddenly crop up in the loads of clothing needed to be cleaned at least once a week. If you're like me, you're also determined to do it all as cheaply and chemical-free as possible.

Let's start with the heavy hitters when it comes to home toxins: fabric softeners and dryer sheets. Got your attention? Most people add fabric softeners and dryer sheets to their laundry, and most people never give it a second thought. We all want soft, static-free clothing that smells good, right? But if you really knew what was going on in these products, you'd ditch them faster than you can say "static cling." For starters, the host of chemicals in your fabric softeners and dryer sheets are horribly toxic. Try benzyl acetate, which is linked to pancreatic cancer. Or benzyl alcohol, an upper respiratory tract irritant. How about ethanol, which can cause central nervous system disorders? A-terpineol, another respiratory irritant, which can also cause fatal edema and central nervous system damage. Ethyl Acetate is a narcotic on the EPA's Hazardous Waste list. Camphor can cause central nervous system disorders.

Chloroform, that stuff they use in movie crimes to knock people out, is neurotoxic, anesthetic, and carcinogenic. Linalool is a narcotic that can also cause central nervous system disorders. And pentane is a chemical that should not be inhaled. If we piece all these chemicals together, not only do we have a recipe for bodily damage and environmental risk, we have a massive stink. Which is why producers of these laundry items have to add all the strong fragrances.

  I'll admit, I can get on my natural soap box when it comes to fabric softeners and dryer sheets. After having given up on them many years ago, along with other highly fragranced items, though, I'll tell you the biggest thing I've noticed: My sense of smell has become akin to that of a wolf. I can smell people coming from a long way off, especially if they use the dryer sheets. It's a game with my husband and myself: Name the dryer sheet. Laugh all you like, but I've realized over the years how much my nose was inundated with artificial smells, in particular those found in laundry products, and how much they deadened my sense of smell. I now walk past people's houses when the dryer is going and... I gag. I can smell the chemicals that once I could not. And I definitely notice the effects on asthma if I spend more than five minutes in someone's house who likes to use the really strong dryer sheets, or, heaven forbid, the fragrance plugins which are another major culprit. It makes me wonder what those same chemicals would do to a baby if a baby was surrounded, swaddled, and wrapped in fabric softener residue every single day and night of their new lives. This is the perfect place to start a chemical-free household: Ditch the fabric softener, toss the dryer sheets.

For an alternative to fabric softeners, dryer sheets, and even bleach, try some vinegar. It also kills germs and bacteria, which ordinary laundry soaps don't do. Don't worry, your shirts will not smell like a tossed salad when you're done. The vinegar odor is completely gone when the laundry comes out of the dryer. I usually use about ¾ cup per load, which is probably more than necessary. Again, a cheap solution, so if you use a little extra like me, you won't break the bank. Another trick I enjoy is to keep a cheaper brand of pure essential oil, such as lavender or rosemary, near the washing machine. I add several drops to the rinse cycle cup to make my laundry fresh. It also kills germs and bacteria.

If you just can't live without fragrant clothing, you can make your own dryer sheets by putting dried herbs such as lavender, rose petals, rosemary, or sage into tightly tied bundles. Use an old sock and tie the end off after filling it with herbs, then toss it into the dryer with your clothing. You can reuse this bundle until the fragrance is gone. Or apply a few drops of essential oil to boost the scent. The good news is, these fragrances will not overpower and will be safe for baby.

If you live in a temperate climate, line drying will certainly cut back on the electric bill and give you wonderful smelling laundry to boot. Even in the dead of winter, we're often seen in our back yard hanging blankets and sheets all over our deck railings. The UV light of sunshine is also a terrific way to kill germs. Another great thing about sunshine: It's totally free!

For an alternative to laundry soap, try borax. I know, it's supposed to be an addition to your laundry soap, right? But what most people don't realize is that on its own this powerful little natural mineral is able to bind itself to dirt, dissolving it. It also softens the water and creates its own peroxide, which in turn gives you whiter whites, and it's safe for soaking cloth diapers in (½ cup in a diaper pail of warm water) and can make the diapers more absorbent. Talk about cheap! Around here, a box of the 20 Muleteam Borax runs about $3.50. I have a front-loading washer which requires less detergent, so one of these boxes lasts me quite a while.

Ways to clean your home naturally abound. If you try a natural solution and it doesn't work for you, don't give up. I've tried and tested many, many solutions and thrown more out the window than I've kept. But I'm always pleasantly surprised to find something natural that's more effective than the usual expensive store-bought solutions. It becomes a fulfilling challenge. The best part? You feel more self-sufficient and you know you've got a safe, true clean in your house.

The Impossible Task of Clean: Organizational Tips

Are you drowning in unfolded laundry? Has your kitchen counter become lost? Are your dust bunnies threatening the dog? If so, there's a good chance you are an overwhelmed parent. I, too, often struggle from a bad case of housecleaning blues. But over the years I've come up with solutions to dig my way out of the clutter.

Lists Aren't Just for Obsessive Compulsives

Although I have often swayed from my own advice, the one bit I keep returning to, the one that really works, is the list on the refrigerator. I have found that making a list with only one housecleaning task assigned per each day of the week would make it a lot easier to keep up on the usual vacuuming, laundry, and general cleaning. I personally find this helpful as long as I do my one chore each day. Saturday is no longer the clean-till-you-drop day. And when, say, Monday comes around, I know that's when I vacuum. If the ironing isn't done, too bad. Ironing isn't for Monday. I'm off the hook!

Pickup and Drop-off

Whenever you pass through a room, look for something to take with you. For instance, you're on your way to the baby's room and you notice a baby sock (why do those end up everywhere?) on the coffee table. Take it with you. You're that much further ahead. I am home all day, and I move a lot unless I'm chained to my computer typing a mean streak. I should amend this: I move a lot when I'm avoiding typing a mean streak. I have noticed that when I stick to this tip of picking up and dropping off, it's amazing what gets put away, and what I've overlooked for an embarrassingly long period of time. (Like that 9-volt battery on the end table.

What was that for, anyway?)

If you live in a two-story house, you can use a couple of bins, one for upstairs and one for down, to help you get things back in place. While you're upstairs and moving around, dump as much downstairs stuff in the bin as you can. The next time you head down, you'll be able to move a lot more odds and ends back to where they belong.

Bag It Up

One I find great joy in doing is hanging a disposable bag on a door handle somewhere in the middle of the house or where I pass by most often. When I find things to throw away, in it goes. It's amazing what can be tossed in the course of an afternoon while moving from room to room. It's a cleansing, purging sort of thing.

Chill Out and Dump

Every time you get in the refrigerator, try and find something, just one thing, that needs to be dumped. If your fridge is overflowing with outdated and questionable substances, the idea of a complete cleaning is probably overwhelming. But tossing one item each time you open the door will make a dent in a hurry! Before you know it, your fridge will be clean and without even rolling up your sleeves. This tip also works for other things like the junk drawer, your makeup drawer, closets, and any other place things are often tossed out of view.

Sink In and Prepare

Every sink in your house should have a few cleaning items under it for quick cleaning. Things to have at the ready would be: a small spray bottle of vinegar and water for glass, chrome, and counter tops; a sponge; baking soda or your favorite natural cleansing powder; a roll of paper towel or a few cleaning cloths; a microfiber cloth for dry-buffing sink fixtures. Now you don't have to run from one end of the house to the other to find the ever-elusive cleanser. And when you happen to notice the sink is looking questionable, your gear is right there. Saves lots of time and energy. This one tip has rescued me more than once. Imagine guests dropping in to see your new baby. You know that bathroom sink is growing fur, but you can't exactly excuse yourself and run past them with cleaning products under your arms. "Pardon me, I must scrape the toothpaste off the counter before you use the facilities." Now you can use the excuse you must use the restroom, then spray around a little and wipe it all down with a paper towel. Voila! You become one of those people that others secretly think always has a clean house.

These sorts of tips sound great and they're encouraging, but they're even better if you commit to them. Busy parents simply don't have time to do major cleaning overhauls, especially with a baby to care for. With a small amount of effort, you can save yourself from running in frustrating circles later. Who knows? You might even be able to knock off a few of those mutant dust bunnies.

Natural Beauty for Mom

Pregnancy is probably one of the most intense ways to discover all the things you do to yourself that you probably shouldn't. Suddenly, every bite of fast food, every trip to the nail salon, every dab of moisturizer comes under scrutiny. I remember being keenly aware that whatever my body absorbed, so did my baby. It was an eye opening experience, and much of how I live today is due to those nine months of self-questioning.

For many moms, breast feeding follows pregnancy; hence, more questions, perhaps more worries and doubts. But just because you've had a baby doesn't mean you can't pamper yourself. Quite the opposite is true; now is the time to give yourself little boosts whenever you can.

Making your own beauty products doesn't have to be difficult or time consuming or expensive. With just a few ingredients, you can have money saving products that often rival (or even blow away) store bought beauty supplies. While my books Beauty Gone Wild and Hair Gone Wild go into greater detail, including natural skin care and hair coloring, I've included a few of my favorite easy beauty tips here. They're chemical free, they work, and pregnant and nursing moms can enjoy them with no worries.

Natural Skin Care & DIY Health Products

Homemade Body Oils

Whether it's cold and dry, or it's day-in-the-sun weather, body oils are nourishing and easy to prepare. I use them daily instead of moisturizer during the coldest, driest times of the year and after a day at the beach. Add the right essential oils and you've got custom made skin!

What you'll need:

A choice of oils. I often use sweet almond oil, but other favorites are avocado and olive oil. While the almond and avocado soak into the skin faster, olive is much heavier. If you've got dry skin or if you live in a desert climate, try some olive oil.

A selection of essential oils. The blend I use most of the time is a mix of patchouli and ylang ylang, which is an amazing combination to eliminate wrinkles and reverse sun damage. These really do work, especially if you're able to get some good quality oils.

A 4-ounce bottle. I like to reuse bottles and jars for this, preferably something with a small opening. Order something beautiful or reuse something you have on hand. In my experience, there's always a good container somewhere under the bathroom cupboard filled with something you don't like, anyway. Just make sure it is cleaned out thoroughly and doesn't smell of something else before you add your oils.

So, which essential oils will you choose? I've provided a partial list below.

Essential Oils by Skin Type:

Acne: Bergamot, cedarwood, chamomile, Clary sage, clove, eucalyptus, frankincense, geranium, juniper, lavender, lemon, lemongrass, marjoram, myrtle, patchouli, petitgrain, ravensara, rosemary, rosewood, sage, sage lavender, sandalwood, spearmint, tea tree, thyme, vetiver, yarrow.

Cellulite: Basil, cedarwood, cumin, cypress, fennel, geranium, grapefruit, juniper, lavender, lemon, lime, orange, oregano, patchouli, rosemary, rosewood, sage, spikenard (increases metabolism to burn fat), tangerine (dissolves), thyme.

Dry: Atlas cedar, carrot seed, chamomile, davana, geranium, jasmine, lavender, lemon, neroli, patchouli, rosewood, sandalwood, spikenard, vetiver, ylang ylang.

Mature/Wrinkles: carrot seed, cistus, Clary sage, cypress, elemi, fennel seed, frankincense, galbanum, geranium, helichrysum, jasmine, lavender, lemon, lime, myrrh, neroli, orange, oregano, patchouli (prevents wrinkles), rose, rosehips (slows wrinkles), rosemary (verbene type), rosewood (slows wrinkles), sandalwood, spikenard, thyme, ylang ylang.

Instructions:

Pour your carrier oil (almond, avocado, or olive) into your container. Then add either a single or a combination of essential oils, about 10 to 12 drops of essential oil per every ounce of carrier you use. For example, if you've chosen a 4-ounce bottle, you'd use a total of no more than 48 drops of essential oils.

Cap and shake before use.

That's it! Enjoy healthy, glowing skin year round. I'm sure you'll notice a difference in the feel and look of your skin after you've given your natural homemade face and body oils a try.

One-Ingredient Skin Care Tricks

You don't need to stock up on essential oils and special ingredients if you don't want to, however. If you take a moment to look in your kitchen cupboard, we can hook you up with some serious facial products. Let's start with cleansing, shall we?

Baking soda is a fantastic exfoliant. Using a small amount, maybe ⅛ of a teaspoon, massage it gently onto damp skin. Rinse thoroughly. Use it once or twice a week to keep your skin smooth, but not every day. Its exfoliating power is a bit much for that, and you could irritate your skin if you overdo it.

Now for your cleanser. I always keep a bottle of honey in my bathroom, preferably the little bear because he's cheery and makes me feel better when I'm tired and want to hurl heavy objects at the mirror. After you exfoliate, or whenever your skin needs extra moisturizing, rub about a teaspoon to a tablespoon of honey on slightly damp skin and allow it to sit for up to five minutes. Rinse with water. Honey is water soluble and rinses off cleanly, but I'd advise putting your hair back for this. While honey is nice as a hair conditioner, it kind of fails as hair gel. You can use the honey every day if you like. Besides moisturizing better than any face mask I've ever spent hard earned money on, it rocks at removing fine lines and wrinkles, and it reverses sun damage too. It takes only one use to see and feel a difference in your skin.

After a thorough cleanse, it's nice to follow up with a good moisturizer. When you're taking care of an infant, you need quick and simple. Try coconut oil. You can use it all over the body, not just the face, and it smells wonderful. Be sure to get a good organic jar of it, and make sure to check the expiration date. Coconut oil should smell like coconuts. If it doesn't, take it back and get another jar. The difference is worth it.

Homemade Toothpaste

While it may sound like a complicated process, learning how to make your own natural homemade toothpaste couldn't be easier. Chances are, you already have some of the ingredients rattling around your kitchen; and if you don't, they're easy to find and inexpensive.

Here's the recipe:

2 Tbs. baking soda

2 Tbs. organic coconut oil

½ tsp. organic raw honey

3 to 5 drops essential oil such as

spearmint, peppermint, cinnamon or clove

Just a dash of sea salt or kosher salt

Dump all these ingredients into a bowl and smash it with a fork, mushing the coconut oil into the mixture until it looks just like – well, just like toothpaste. Scrape all the well-mixed paste into a glass container with a tight fitting lid and use just as you would your regular, expensive, and not-so-natural paste.

That's it! You've just learned how to make a natural and homemade toothpaste at a fraction of the cost of store-bought brands and it's safe enough for even the youngest teeth in the family.

Safe & Natural Deodorant Solutions

Research has shown that virtually all breast cancer tumors contain parabens, a common ingredient in underarm deodorants and beauty products. Another common deodorant ingredient, aluminum chloride, may also contribute to breast cancer risks. Since we know chemicals put under the arms can travel to the breast, it's best to take precautions when deodorizing. It's also important to realize that when we use antiperspirants, we are essentially blocking the body's ability to release toxins through the lymph nodes that reside there. And keeping toxins trapped in the body is never a good thing.

There are several natural remedies I can offer you. Try them all until you find the one that works best for you.

Baking soda again enters the picture. Using just a pinch, rub it into your damp palms then under the arms. Reapply as needed.

Lemon juice is another effective deodorant. A squirt of lemon juice under each arm is enough to keep you feeling fresh throughout the day. You can keep a small spray bottle of the juice handy for reapplication.

I also enjoy throwing together this simple recipe for underarm spray that is both refreshing and wonderfully scented. Prepare a tea of coriander by steeping two teaspoons of the seeds in a cup of boiling water for about 30 to 40 minutes. Strain out the seeds, then wait for the tea to fully cool. Add 10 drops of lemongrass essential oil and five drops of lavender essential oil. Place the mixture in a spray bottle and spray under arms as needed.

A Final Word

This is just the beginning of your baby's natural, beautiful life. You're giving her a start that, while she won't remember all the efforts you took to make homemade baby food or preparing diaper salve, she'll have the health and the good eating habits to prove you did it. And you'll always know.

As a final bit of advice, don't stress out. Parents who are conscious of living a healthier, greener life can easily feel overwhelmed with it all. It's impossible to be a parent and not feel the weight of responsibility in every aspect of our children's lives. Just take things one step at a time. Some things you'll get right. Other things you won't. And that's okay. Remember, the journey to good health and chemical-free living isn't an instantaneous leap. It's one step followed by another and another. Someday you'll look back and wonder how you got where you are! And your children will have been raised seeing you make the effort. From there, they can continue the same forward direction.

Bibliography

Bove, Mary, N.D. An Encyclopedia of Natural Healing for Children & Infants. New York, NY: McGraw-Hill, 2001.

Candee, Andrea. Gentle Healing for Baby & Child. New York, NY: Gallery Books, 2010.

Dodt, Colleen K. Natural Baby Care. North Adams, MA: Storey Books, 1997.

Gladstar, Rosemary. Herbal Remedies for Children's Health. North Adams, MA: Storey Books, 1999.

Greene, Diana S. 79 Ways to Calm a Crying Baby. New York, NY: Pocket, 1988.

Hogg, Tracy and Blau, Melinda. Secrets

of the Baby Whisperer. New York, NY: Ballantine Books, 2001.

Karp, Harvey, M.D. The Happiest Baby on the Block. New York, NY: Bantam, 2008.

Kemper, Kathy J., M.D., M.P.H. The Holistic Pediatrician (2nd ed.) New York, NY: Harper Perennial, 2002.

Liu, Henry C. Chinese Natural Cures: Traditional Methods for Remedy and Prevention. New York, NY: Black Dog & Leventhal Publishers, 2006.

Liu, Henry C. Traditional Chinese Medicine: An Authoritative and Comprehensive Guide. Laguna Beach, CA: Basic Health Publications, 2005.

O'Mara, Peggy. Natural Family Living. New York, NY: Simon & Schuster, 2000.

About the Author

Diane Kidman studied herbalism with the Southwest School of Botanical Medicine and continues to study through real-life practice. Her focus is on teaching others to incorporate herbalism into their everyday lives, while living a more natural and chemical-free life. She is often found picking and ingesting all manner of weeds and leaves.

You can find Diane's other books on herbalism, health, and natural beauty on her Author Page at Amazon.

Printed in Great Britain
by Amazon